NICE GIRLS DON'T DRINK

NICE GIRLS DON'T DRINK

Stories of Recovery

SARAH HAFNER

BERGIN & GARVEY

New York • Westport, Connecticut • London

Library of Congress Cataloging-in-Publication Data

Nice girls don't drink : stories of recovery / [compiled by] Sarah
  Hafner.
      p.   cm.
   Includes bibliographical references and index.
   ISBN 0-89789-246-1 (alk. paper). — ISBN 0-89789-247-X (pbk. :
alk. paper)
    1. Women alcoholics—United States—Interviews. 2. Women—United
States—Drug use—Case studies. 3. Narcotic addicts—United States—
Interviews.   I. Hafner, Sarah.
HV5137.N53   1992
362.29'082—dc20   91-18924

British Library Cataloguing in Publication Data is available.

Library of Congress Catalog Card Number: 91-18924
ISBN: 0-89789-246-1
     0-89789-247-X (pbk.)

First published in 1992

Bergin & Garvey, One Madison Avenue, New York, NY 10010
An imprint of Greenwood Publishing Group, Inc.

Printed in the United States of America

The paper used in this book complies with the
Permanent Paper Standard issued by the National
Information Standards Organization (Z39.48-1984).

10 9 8 7 6 5 4 3 2 1

Copyright Acknowledgments

My father, an enlightened spirit,
believed in man.
My grandfather, a fervent Hasid,
believed in God.
The one taught me to speak, the other to sing.
Both loved stories.
And when I tell mine, I hear their voices.
Whispering from beyond the silenced storm,
they are what links the survivor to their memory.

—Elie Wiesel,
Souls on Fire

This book is ... by its very nature, about violence,
to the spirit as well as to the body.

—Studs Terkel,
Working

For Dr. Richard J. Maher and
Dr. Jay M. Pomerantz
and for my family

Contents

**Marty
Mann**

214

I saw red when I saw the word God. But there on the page, where it says, "We cannot afford anger," the words were clear, and in white.

*Name has been changed.

Acknowledgments

I would like to thank Deborah Klaum, who believed in this book from the beginning, and Sophy Craze, my editor at Bergin & Garvey. I also want to thank Studs Terkel, Bruce Grant, Dr. Jean Kirkpatrick, Frank Wright, Christine Thibault, Barbara Rivest, Carmelina LoRusso, Marianne Mackay, Donald Dunkenberg, Victor De-Michele, David Hiller, Neil Hammer, The National Council On Alcoholism and Drug Dependence, Hermine Deso, Karl Dunkenberg, John Rozum, Mary Connor Ralph, Ken Forfia, Thomas Ripa, Bruce Marcille, Everett and Pamela Hafner, Talvi Laev, Denise Van Acker, John Lewis, James Sawyer, and John Dooley. Both John Bowman and Leslie Dunkenberg helped me edit the final version. I am indebted to my sister, Katie Hafner, who encouraged me to write this. I don't know how to thank the women who had the courage to speak up; without them this book would not have been possible.

Introduction

What does it feel like to be a woman in America who is an alcoholic? What did the first drink feel like? How does a woman's drinking affect her children, her husband, her lover, her work? And how did she come to stop?

This book attempts to answer those questions through women's own stories. It offers them a place of their own, a place where they can speak for themselves instead of having someone speak for them, or to them. Its pages contain a series of interviews with recovering alcoholic women. Unless they have chosen otherwise, they have kept their anonymity.

I embarked on this project in part because of my own experience, but mostly because I was in search of women I could admire. As a recovering alcoholic I was frustrated by the lack of alcoholic histories told by women.

So I set out with my tape recorder, sitting for the better part of a day in a stranger's home, on the phone, or in a coffee shop, just listening to women speak. Some of the stories poured out in an uninterrupted stream; others were halting, difficult to elicit. All were riveting. They were at once deeply personal, thoughtful, enlightening, hopeful, frightening, depressing, and humorous. These stories are, at least in part, reconstructions of events told to the women by others—spouses, neighbors, friends, the police, their own children. Periods of blackout are impossible to recall. Few of these stories have fairy-tale endings, largely because recovering from alcoholism requires a quiet surrender—acquiescence. Trying to conquer alcoholism with brute force—the way we tackle other problems—hastens its progression.

In conceiving this book, I was convinced that there were thousands of women whose personal stories of recovery would prove just as compelling and inspiring as hours spent poring over self-help books. I felt that the identification process many women experience in Alcoholics Anonymous could also be felt in a book.

Recovery usually begins when a woman hears a story similar to her own. Therefore I chose women from varied backgrounds and professions. Housewives, sales clerks, counselors, and artists are here together telling of a disease that transcends distinctions of class, education, and culture. "I was looking at the speaker," said Jane, thinking about one of her first Alcoholics Anonymous meetings. "Her nails were almond shaped and perfect, her hair was lovely. . . . The rage was unbelievable. I thought, 'You have never been where I have been.' Then I noticed as she went to light a cigarette that her hand was trembling and in that moment I became interested in another human being. I think that's when my recovery began."

To most people sobriety means simply "not drinking." The women in this book feel differently. Denise, for instance, said, "I learned that I am worthy of love. That it's okay to love myself." Margaret said, "Before I came into A.A., or got sober, I was some sort of Buddhist freak, always searching for God in drugs and alcohol. Now everything is being explained." While Karen said, "The biggest lesson I've learned is that sobriety is a process. I'm always amazed when speakers in Alcoholics Anonymous say, 'A.A. gave me back my life.' I never had a life."

It was an effort for me to stay in the background, to let these women emerge. Instinctively I knew better than to keep my responses to myself but I deleted them in the finished versions. The women inevitably asked, "Do you know what I mean?" or "Can you believe it?" There were times I identified so strongly with them it terrified me.

At times I felt that I was trespassing, invading someone's privacy. Sometimes I had to cancel and reschedule. It was awkward looking at the phone and thinking about how to explain that I had another appointment. These women were taking the time to tell me about their lives, no matter how painful or difficult to remember. Who was more important? I knew I had to take care of myself, but it was never easy to put myself first. Sometimes I simply had too many voices trapped inside my own head and I had to step back.

Given that alcoholism is a disease that accounts for the deaths of nearly one hundred thousand every year, a disease responsible for the majority of suicides and car accidents on any given day, a disease that bullies its victims into believing that they do not, in fact, *have* a disease, it is hard to understand why most doctors don't recognize it. My own physical signs of alcoholism went undiagnosed for almost three years. Because of unbearable stomach pain, I was frequently hospitalized, both in the United States and in England. It didn't matter where I went; the doctors never asked me how much I drank. They all seemed to feel that I was simply nervous. Finally the appropriate test revealed the pain as pancreatitis, one of the first symptoms of alcoholism.

I have always believed that alcoholism flares up in men and women differently. Men are taught that it is an expression of masculinity to drink, while women are abhorred and ostracized if they do the same. A man can drink openly and heavily, and then boast about it. A woman who drinks in public is considered loose and unreliable, not to be trusted to get dinner on the table, to say nothing of holding down a job. Some women tend to turn inward; they stay at home in hiding with their liquor, closing themselves off from a world that judges them harshly, leaving the house only to replenish their stash. They shop at different liquor stores, attempting to remain anonymous. They are afraid of being caught. This makes it harder for a woman to seek help and stay sober. Even in this so-called enlightened society, to admit that she has a problem, to say to a new friend or lover, "I am an alcoholic," usually invites rejection.

Although I did not set out to draw conclusions, similarities among the women began to appear. While drinking, most of these women say they felt different and alone. Because of low self-esteem, they were attracted to abusive relationships. More often than not they come from alcoholic homes. Bruised children, they were becoming abusive parents. Most of them still smoke cigarettes.

I did not use a prepared set of questions. A question I asked in the beginning—"Would you ever pick up a drink or a drug again?"—I forgot about toward the end because the answer was always an emphatic "No." My tape recorder picked up silence, laughter, sobs, a smoker's cough; it didn't discriminate. But my mind did. When I read these stories I saw things that I hadn't noticed in the initial conversations. Checking my original tapes to make sure there were no mistakes, I discovered the written versions were accurate. When a woman received her copy of an interview, she too was often surprised by what she had said. I began to wait for transcriptions with the anticipation one feels while waiting for a roll of film to be developed.

In sobriety I learned that I could do anything. I no longer had drinking as an excuse not to write this book. I had the support of my family and, almost without exception, my friends. The well-meaning husband of a friend told me I had no hope of finding a publisher. "What publisher in his right mind would offer a recovering alcoholic a contract?" I felt as though I'd been stung. But I refused to believe that my past would foretell my future. And so I began advertising for recovering alcoholic women.

I started getting phone calls and letters from women who had heard about the book. Lucy wrote, "I have so many childhood memories of my father's alcoholism. They are clear and painful. My younger brother had a system of closing or opening the drapes depending on my father's state of composure. If I saw the drapes open on my way home from school, I would bring a friend home to play. If they were closed I would return home alone, and, as I walked, prepare myself emotionally for my father's drunken state. I also remember wondering why our kitchen sponges always stank. When I went to visit friends, I would secretly smell their kitchen sponges and wonder why they didn't smell as foul. They smelled like Ivory Liquid. Now I know that the mixture of food, alcohol, and time created the smell. People have told me I should write a book about my childhood. But who, I thought, wants to read about rancid sponges, about standing in a liquor store with your father, begging him to buy a smaller bottle of beer, or the secret meaning of closed drapes? I would. And I am not alone."

This book is about women who have confronted a disease in a society where they are disadvantaged to begin with. Therefore, it is as much about living with an uninvited guest who is here to stay as it is about learning to respect ourselves. Gaining self-respect requires taking responsibility for one's actions; it means learning to say *no* without the nagging concern that the recipient of that simple word might be upset or love us less. It begins with the spark of courage gained from disregarding the way in which others view us, caring instead about how we perceive *ourselves*. While alcohol initially gave us a sense of self-esteem, it eventually robbed us of it altogether. Recovery is, ultimately, about reclaiming dignity, a feeling so alien to most of us while in the final stages of addiction that the fear of losing it keeps us sober.

In most cases, it was helpful—even therapeutic—for the women here to tell their stories into a small machine that would neither criticize nor talk back; it was a way of coming to terms all over again. And it is my hope that it helps others just as much to read the stories, to sit curled up by themselves, pick up the book on impulse and read at random. Part of our ability to survive hinges on our capacity for imagination. Living alone with an imagination can lead to self-destruction. But sharing it in the form of a friendship, or in the pages of a book, alive with the landscape of others, can sustain us.

Part One

Making It Through the Night

Not out of vengeance have I accomplished all my sins, but because something has always been close to dying in my soul, and I've sinned in order to lie down in darkness and find, somewhere in the net of dreams, a new father, a new home.

—William Styron,
Lie Down in Darkness

Jane

Jane has been sober since October 15, 1965. She walked through the doors of Alcoholics Anonymous when she was thirty years old. Because she is a writer and people might recognize her, we discussed anonymity. "Anonymity promotes truth, and truth is the foundation for recovery," she said. A man in A.A. related his impression on hearing her speak: "It was the most profound experience of my sobriety. It felt as though we were all being touched by God's grace. I will never forget it for as long as I live."

I was born in the West Indies. My father was an American aviator. My mother was from Scotland. She came to this country when she was quite young. And alcoholism runs in her side of the family, the way judges and generals do in others.

I was fascinated by drinking and legend has it that I had my first blackout at age six, when I scaled the walls in the kitchen and got a bottle of crème de menthe, which I drank until I lost consciousness. Now, crème de menthe was a real treat, as was ice cream, because, living in the tropics, we didn't have any refrigeration like we have here. The cook would crank the ice cream out and then it would be sprinkled with crème de menthe. I loved the stuff, so that should have been the first sign—to the adults at least—that something was abnormal.

If you saw the movie *Out of Africa*, we lived in a bungalow like that. My father had his own plane and he would whiz in and out, swoop over the house—it was a very idyllic life. And drinking was a lovely ritual. I used to love to sit and listen to the grown-ups. They were fascinating. They were beautiful. They were exciting and had interesting things to say. They would sit on the veranda and the houseboy would pass among them in a sparkling white coat with a tray of tinkling concoctions in glasses. I couldn't wait to grow up and be like them.

My mother was already evolving into her alcoholism. I don't know if my father was an alcoholic or not because he didn't live long enough. He was killed in World War II when he was twenty-nine years old. The day he was killed I was off on a field trip at the zoo. I remember waiting my turn to ride the elephant. Just as I was about to get on I was snatched off, thrown into one of those old woody Ford station wagons, with a woman at the wheel who said nothing to me on the long drive back to our house. We had a police motor-cycle escort. When we got to the house, the media was crawling all over. Reporters, photographers from the New York papers, the Long Island papers, were shoving cameras, flashbulbs—the big old ones—in my face. I was terrified. I asked my mother's older sister what was happening. My aunt grabbed me by the arm, gave me a yank, a real shove, and said, "Stop that." I was crying. She said, "Your father's been killed. You'll make your mother cry." I was seven years old.

I was thrown onto the couch next to my mother and my photo-graph appeared all over the New York papers the next day. *"Here's little Jane: she doesn't know her father is dead."* I think the media was just as ghoulish and tacky then as they are now.

That began the business of no expectations from an adult. That you had to be tough, you had to be strong. A lot of it was that Scottish-British stiff upper lip stuff. No one comforted me, no one talked to me about my loss. One day an attractive, golden, exciting man was in my life and the next day he was gone. There was a memorial service, but the belief in those days was that children should not go to funerals. So I never even had that, that rite of passage. I was just waiting for some sort of narcotic to ease my pain, but I wasn't drinking at that point. I'm sure if it had occurred to me, I would have. It didn't occur to me there might be magic in those glasses.

We also had a home in the States, we'd go back and forth, and when the war broke out I was quite small. We left everything behind, which we'd done many times before, but I didn't know we weren't ever going back. Life changed dramatically. It changed for everyone with the war.

My mother remarried. She was very young, still in her twenties. She married a guy who was the son of an alcoholic but he himself was not an alcoholic. However, he was obviously seriously affected by the disease. He was the antithesis of my father. He was brutal and violent and abusive physically and verbally. So I learned early to shut down and be quiet. I never knew what would set him off. Of course I'd try very hard to be good so as not to provoke this behavior, this violence which was so alien to me. He went into the navy and we moved to Washington, D.C. That was a lot of fun because there were billions of kids. We were living in a barracks-type situation at first. I spent all my time outside running like a little hooligan. We would reenact World War II in the construction trenches. Now the drinking became more intense among the grown-ups. People were going away and never coming back. But it didn't have that same magical kind of—unreal romantic quality that it had before. Now a more desperate kind of thing went with it.

During the war my mother and my stepfather had a child, my half-sister. One day after returning to Long Island, as I was preparing to go to school, my mother suggested I not wear what I was going to put on, and said put on . . . which were my dressy clothes. I said, "But why?" and she said, "You're not going to school today, we're going over to Mineola, to the courthouse. You're being adopted." I was not consulted and you have to remember that during this era, this period, children had no rights whatsoever. The tenet that children should be seen and not heard was very much in place.

You were being adopted by your stepfather?

Yes. And so this was done. The judge leaned over afterwards, a kindly old man, and said, "How do you like your new name?" and I whispered under my breath, I mean I was seething inside, and I said, "I hate it." My mother was furious. How could I say a thing like that? There was no consideration for what my feelings on the matter might have been. This was done so we all could be a family. You see, they had a child together and their thinking, their rationale was well meant. What I felt, and it's an issue many women feel, was that my identity—in that moment—had been stripped from me without any warning.

When the war was over we came back to Long Island, which was where the home my father had built was. Shortly after that, my mother and her second husband decided to move to Connecticut and bought some land up in this area. I was about eleven. We moved and I was put into a girls' country day school, a prep school.

We were well-to-do. But all things are relative and I was meeting girls who came from enormously wealthy families. In the old society we had been exciting and dramatic and well off. Now we were on the other end of the spectrum. I'd also become withdrawn and shy and I remember booze was always around the house. I hated school. It was run on the British system. We all received excellent educations as far as academics went, but it was so painful and so excruciating that I remember walking—when I was about twelve—into the pantry and just reaching for a bottle. I believe it was scotch. I poured myself a drink. I drank it and that began the pattern that continued throughout my life. I drank daily. I drank in the morning and I drank for effect at twelve. If I ever drank socially it was in the fraction of a second it took for the alcohol to pass through my lips and into my system.

So I drank daily. I drank alone and I drank in the morning. It was my magical elixir. It relieved the pain, the psychic pain that I was experiencing. It allowed me to pass for normal. I used to have a drink every day before school. What's interesting is, it was a tiny school; there were only eight in my class, but no one picked up on this. I guess it didn't occur to people back then that a child could be drinking. This was in the late forties, early fifties. Apparently I didn't reek of booze. That came later, when it was just oozing out of my pores. The stench was in my clothes; it was disgusting. While this was going on my mother was deteriorating very rapidly. She died at the age of forty-eight of toxic encephalopathy, which is the medical term for wet brain. She was seeing many doctors at the time. Typically of doctors then and I think still today, the physicians would look at her and perceive her as a victim of her own emotions. In fact, if anything, they would say, "Unwind and relax with a little drink."

When I was seventeen and ready to graduate from prep school, there'd been no real thought or plan given to what I would do once I graduated. Yet I was being told things, you know, the business of the high expectations, but the expectations were never defined. It was always, "Well, you could do better, you're not doing well enough." At the same time, my mother would say to me, "You're your father's daughter." There was yet another expectation because he was so remarkable. And it was expected that I would up and do something utterly fantastic. But there was never any discussion of how I would go about doing this. It was just assumed that somehow I would evolve full-blown into something spectacular. So I drank to ease those pressures and that pain. I began to panic and thought, "Well, all my friends are going away to college," and I was told that I was far too stupid to even consider doing that, yet there was no alternate plan given. Not even "go and learn to type" or anything. Meanwhile, my best friend, or all my best friends, were going off to one of the seven sisters, Wellesley, Holyoke, Vassar, whatever. So I decided I would go to Paris. I proceeded to get a job and earn the money to go because I knew if I went I would have to pay my own way. I never asked for anything because any time I did all hell would break loose.

Meanwhile, one particular friend, who was also, I now realize, a child alcoholic, was all set to go off to college. Unlike me, she had her full set of parents, a seemingly terrific lifestyle, and was incredibly gifted intellectually. We first met when we were about twelve, at prep school. We would spend weekends together and we would write novels. I had my mother's old Royal portable, she had a Remington. We wrote steamy sagas about sex, about the West, about dynasties; things about which we knew absolutely nothing. My mother never saved any of this stuff, which is too bad. What's interesting is that an English teacher at school took pity on me, I guess, along with a couple of the other lost souls. We would meet in the little garret rooms where the teachers lived and have wine and cheese parties after school. No one thought anything of that either, that there was something untoward about serving wine and cheese to thirteen- and fourteen-year-old girls. Of course, we were drinking like ladies; we weren't sitting there swilling it. But I could never get enough. My eyes would always be fixated on the bottle. It was the magic. My whole drinking career was based on hopes.

I never got drunk. I could drink everybody under the table. They used to call me hollow-body. This went on for quite a while. Meanwhile, my mother was becoming sicker and sicker and crazier and crazier as a result of her alcoholism. My hatred of her was entering a whole new dimension. As an adult woman I can look back at that period, when she would sort of passively stand by while my step-father heaped abuse and physical violence on me, and see that she had no choice. When you're young, you interpret that as abandonment: that he must be right or I must deserve that kind of behavior. Part of the system of recovery has been unraveling all of that, developing a fuller understanding, not only of my own disease but of her disease and how my stepfather was affected. It was truly a recipe for catastrophe. But I really developed a bitter hatred for my mother, for what she had become, and vowed early on that I would never be like her. Of course, you know what happened, not only was I like her, I was worse. She was a housewife sneaking her gins from under the kitchen sink, and I went on to become a woman alone in a major metropolis. While I'm not demeaning her suffering or humiliation, or the degradation I know she felt, I lived it out and acted it out in a much more dangerous fashion than she ever did. Just by virtue of the physical circumstances.

Such as driving a car?

Driving, or doing things with anyone in order to get a drink. I can remember being in a phone booth in what is now called the East Village, in those days it was called the Bowery—in New York—with nine guys beating on the door trying to get at me. I remember having a flash of terror that my mother didn't raise me to be in this situation, but not being able to help it. So, at seventeen, in my senior year of school, having worked and saved money, I announced that I was going to Paris when I graduated. My stepfather said, "Pass the potatoes," and that's how that news was greeted. But as time went by they all took it as a fait accompli. They never said, "Will you need money?" or "What are you going to do once you get there?" It was assumed that I was probably going to go there to study art because I had a mild talent for drawing. But what I really wanted to do was write. This was something that I didn't mention to anyone. I just thought, well, I'm not educated enough, I'm not good enough. I accepted the art thing because it didn't mean that much to me and if I failed, it wouldn't matter. My parents did arrange for me to live with the mother of one of their friends.

I got to Paris, I sailed over. I had a one-way boat ticket and a small amount of cash, that was it. I had no idea what I would really do, I was not enrolled in any kind of school or studio. It was just assumed that I would magically evolve eventually into a stupendous painter in Paris. I would live with this nice mother of the friend in Westport. Mme O. had a flat in the 14th Arrondissement of Paris. She spoke no English and although I'd had French in school it was hardly conversational.

The first thing I was given was a bottle of white stuff and a little cold supper. I went out on the balcony with this bottle. The woman I was staying with was in her seventies and a professional funeral goer. It didn't matter if she knew the people, she just went to the funerals. When I arrived she was off at an engagement and had asked a daughter-in-law to greet me.

What was the little white bottle?

It was Calvados—white lightning—not the stuff you buy commercially. The cache had been buried before the German occupation by Mme O.'s brother and it was discovered when some of the bottles began to blow up. Flore handed me the bottle. This woman had never seen an American woman before, and was terrified. She said, "Au revoir," slammed on her hat, and lurked off into the night. So here I am, I'm in Paris, I'm seventeen years old, it's the autumn, it's October, I've got this bottle of hooch, it's been indicated I can have it. I uncorked it and I drank it and I thought I had died and gone to heaven. It literally blew the toenails off my feet.

I did try to paint. I located a studio run by a very eccentric Frenchwoman who took me on. She realized I had no money, that I was not a rich American. She took pity on me and let me teach the younger pupils, even though I didn't know what I was doing. I would drink to go to the studio, and I drank all day long, wine and so on.

That winter there was a nasty rape that occurred in the cellar of the building I lived in. It was supposed to be my romantic losing my virginity night. It turned out to be a violent and terrible assault. And of course in those days, you didn't tell anyone because the assumption was you were always automatically at fault. That you had asked for it. The rape was not by the young man that I was seeing but a crazed Marxist who lived in the building. I was treated by a physician and given drugs which you could get over the counter there. Mme O. said, "Oh, here, have a drink." Brandy. So there I am, taking a strong narcotic, plus the brandy, wafting in and out of reality.

Apparently in a blackout, now I'm nineteen, I agreed to come home, to work for an illustrator. And I have no memory of accepting this job. The next thing I knew, I came to when I was on the *Queen Elizabeth*, sailing for New York. I was sailing tourist. There had been three other women in the cabin with me who asked to be moved. I realize now that I was having my first case of withdrawal and probably DTs. When I came to I had a stale cheese sandwich on my chest and the cabin was empty. I didn't know how the sandwich got there, or where I was, and was finally able to piece together that I was on the ship. All I could think was, I must be going home, and I crawled up to the deck, going up for air. I was deathly ill, withdrawing from alcohol. I weighed 180 pounds of alcoholic bloat. I'm five feet eight. It was a terrible crossing. I staggered off the ship.

It was pre-hippie days, but my hair was hanging down to my knees. I was some kind of physical portent of what was yet to come. I spent an absolutely miserable year. I had no money, I had to work off my passage. The minute my commitment to the illustrator was up, I went to New York.

Having no skills whatsoever, and some small experience in summer stock, I went into the theater. The next decade, my twenties, was spent—in looking back—working with some truly remarkable people. Of course, the fears were increasing. I would drink whenever I could. People brought me wine or booze as I could never scrounge enough money to buy my own. My drinking wasn't out of control, simply because I couldn't afford it.

Who were the people you were working with?

Well, there were playwrights, there were producers, there were actors. One of whom . . . I don't know if you saw the PBS series on the Group Theater last year, but Harold Clurman was one of the founders of the Group Theater. Elia Kazan was in it, Lee Strasberg, Harold's ex-wife, Stella Adler, the great acting teacher who is still teaching in addition to being a great director. . . . Harold was also a theater critic. Harold liked me a lot and I was his assistant on a couple of plays. One was an all-star revival of Shaw's *Heartbreak House* with an English cast. Harold would try to talk to me, sensing something was really radically wrong. You have to remember, in those days, in the arts or in any creative field, the most bizarre and unconscionable behavior was tolerated as being part of the creative process. Yet Harold knew better. I remember during the pre-Broadway tryouts of *Heartbreak House*, Harold took me to dine in a very posh club in Washington, D.C. He knew everyone there—Supreme Court justices, senators, congressmen, and you know, people who were important in the government at that time. That was in the late fifties, and I was in my early twenties. I remember Harold saying to me . . . I remember him looking me in the eye, and waving his cigar and saying, "My darling, life is a losing proposition, so why not make the most of it?" But my fears then were that . . . if he really knew me, he would know what I knew, that there was no one inside. So I was running as any alcoholic will, people-pleasing all over the place, covering up the fact that I didn't know what I was doing and drinking more to relieve the anxiety, the fear and the pain. Just getting caught in the vortex.

I lived a twenty-four-hour program, even then, of drinking and drugging. All my money went for drinking. I rarely bought clothes, I would just try and keep myself decent. I rarely ate. My weight would fluctuate between concentration camp thin and bloated, alcoholic edema. Now I was starting to develop real physical problems. I was beginning to hear things and I wasn't sure if they were really being said. So the way I dealt with that was, have another drink and just be quiet. This was interpreted as great profundity, since the quieter I became, the deeper they thought I was. I would come out with these non sequiturs every now and then, usually in response to an hallucination. And people would run around for days pondering what it meant. I mean, it was just crazy. The wonder is that I didn't die. But I kept on and in 1960, my mother *did* die.

I remember speaking at an A.A. meeting when I first moved back to Connecticut, saying that I had never been married or had children that I knew of. Everyone fell out of their chairs. Someone came up to me and said, "I've heard of long and intense blackouts, but you mean that, don't you?" And I said, "Absolutely." I really did. My blackouts really were that long. I wasn't losing hours, I was losing

days, sometimes weeks and months of my life that I couldn't account
for. And of course, that made the need—increased the need—to drink
to eliminate those fears.

Anyway, I was introduced to a lovely man, who, with his wife,
Audrey Wood, were great agents in their day. They discovered and
represented people like Marlon Brando, Carson McCullers, Ten-
nessee Williams, William Inge, Robert Anderson. This friend of mine
told me Bill Liebling was looking for someone to work with him,
at a big job with a well-known producer who was, and still is, the
biggest, the best, and the most awesome man in the field. So I agreed
to go over and see Bill Liebling. He and Audrey were both very
short, but giants in the theater. They lived in Westport and, as a
child growing up, I had seen them walking around. They were way
out of my ken at the time and it never occurred to me that I would
ever meet either one of them face-to-face.

So meeting Bill Liebling in their pied-à-terre at the Royalton Hotel,
in New York—right across from the Algonquin—blew my mind.
All through the interview, I must have been oozing sweat. Bill kept
saying to me, "You really remind me of Carson McCullers." And
of course I was flabbergasted. Why, Carson McCullers, she's a great
writer—how could I remind him of her? When I sobered up, I realized
Carson McCullers was a raging alcoholic and probably drank herself
to death. The mysterious paralysis she suffered at the end of her life,
when she couldn't get off the bed, before the strokes, was alcoholic
neuropathy. If you read any of the biographies on McCullers, they
show pictures of her at Yaddo where she looks like she's nine years
old, clutching a thermos full of sherry which she drank all day. But
everyone insisted she wasn't an alcoholic, of course, the stigma was
so great. What a loss.

You hadn't met Studs Terkel?

No. That was in recovery. So, anyway, Bill Liebling hired me
either because I reminded him of Carson, or in spite of it. He
was ill, and it was the illness that was to claim his life. But I
was so fogged up, I can't tell you to this day what he died of. I
think it was cancer but I'm not certain. His job was playreader
for this producer who did really magnificent stuff. Bill's job was
to find and develop new plays for him. I was hired but had to

be approved by the producer. I was paralyzed throughout the whole interview, I was so drunk. The only question I can remember him asking me was something about what I wanted in renumeration and I don't recall what my response was. Whatever it was, it was barely subsistence.

So I went to work for him and Bill never came back in and by default I was now, suddenly, playreader to the most prestigious producer on Broadway. He was also a mover and shaker in politics and worked tirelessly in Jack Kennedy's campaign. He had an enormous office. In those days it would be nothing to walk through the reception area and see Adlai Stevenson sitting waiting to see him, Robert Kennedy, or the president of General Dynamics, or Leonard Bernstein, or anybody who was anything. I was in an environment with people who were truly legendary and who most people in their twenties would never meet.

I was tucked in a back room. I sat with a lamp and lots of scripts which I would read and reject, drinking Jack Daniels, the bottle open on my desk; type up my reader reports, and send them up front to Mr. Z. I think, quite frankly, he had forgotten who I was. He had a large office on a whole floor of a building in New York, which he owned. One day I was sitting there with my feet on the desk, I think I was reading *Variety* with a bottle of Jack Daniels, and I felt a presence behind me and I turned around. It was Mr. Z., who, in my deranged way, I had dubbed "The Moose." I had been drawing these little sketches of everyone with moose antlers coming out of their heads. They were very funny and people loved them, and behind his back everybody called him "The Moose." Suddenly, there was this *moose* hovering over me and he said, "You. In my office in forty-five minutes." Well, I was struck sober, and I knew I was going to be fired. I also intuitively knew I was unemployable and so it took all I had to go to his office. Finally I was ushered in. I mean, people who were equal to him in stature would shrivel on that carpet. I'm approaching his desk, and he sat there like God, smoking a wonderful cigar; a very, very good-looking, stately, distinguished man—very imposing. I somehow managed to get my foot stuck in a wastebasket as I made my entrance. He had to get up and help me extricate my foot, which sort of broke the ice. Then he sat back down, and looked at me and said, "Tell me, exactly what is it you do here?" And I said, in a fit of I don't know what, truth, "Not a damn thing," whereupon he roared with laughter and said the magic words: "Why

don't we go have a drink." That was my pattern. Being at the edge
of the abyss, because of my alcoholism, with someone I would never
have met under any normal circumstances and have it all somehow
work in my favor—at least for a while.

It was wild and funny. But it was terrifying, the fear was so
incredible. We went to Trader Vic's, that much I remember, and it
had this horrible, long staircase that you had to navigate to go to
the ladies' room. It was the old Trader Vic's, the original. I had one
of those ghastly drinks where all the fruit and vegetables and um-
brellas and monkeys are climbing out. I must have knocked back
four or five of those. I never just sipped a drink. I could never get
enough. From that first drink, I could never get enough. I was tossing
these things back and went into a horrendous blackout. I have never
had such a hangover as I had the next day. As Marty Mann once
said, "What we call hangovers would have anyone else in intensive
care." The only thing I knew about alcoholism was that if you missed
work on account of your drinking that meant you were an alcoholic
and I was damned if I was going to be one of those. I went to work
the next day and was green around the gills, and he didn't look so
hot himself. I gathered that we also went out to dinner and that
somehow, during the course of this dinner, he heard my life story
or whatever, because within a week he had arranged for me to be
appointed to the National Cultural Center. Now, I was so mokus
that I didn't know what a stupendous honor this was. I'm not sure
of the time frame but I believe I worked running around the country
helping to raise money to build what is now the Kennedy Center
for about two years, I'm not sure. I really mean that. If I had the
nerve, I suppose I could call and ask.

I guess he was getting concerned about my behavior and actions,
or perhaps somebody in Washington said something about my ex-
pense account, because he said to me, "You know, your job was by
presidential appointment." It was called the NCC, the National Cultural Center. Now I'm being told, "Congress can question the NCC
books. This is the taxpayers' money, so you really must not put in
so much for drinking, but your dry cleaning and that sort of thing
is all right." So even though I only had two dresses, I had big dry
cleaning bills for the two dresses, which of course were never cleaned.
I continued on the job. Meanwhile, people had been saying to me
over a period of time that they had been contacted by the FBI, who
wanted to know all about me. You know how you hear in the

program that people think the FBI is outside the door, or tapping their phone? Well, I thought I was imagining all that stuff.

And were you?

No. You needed security clearance for this job and J. Edgar Hoover was still running things in those days. I can't imagine what must be in my dossier. They must have a really wacko file on me. Well, when I heard that, I got so frightened I did what any normal person would do—I quit. I went to work with another producer, a lovely man, who died a classic alcoholic death of one drink, one pill too many, with the phone off the hook, the receiver in his hand in his beautiful little apartment in the Dakota. I went to work for him as associate producer on a play that was an all-time turkey. It opened and closed. Now I was without a job and completely unemployable.

It had gotten really bad. Now I was out of control. Because, you see, I lived on hope. And I lived on hope even though deep down inside I think I knew the booze was doing this. Yet each time I picked up a drink, I lived in hope that it would be the way it once had been. That the magic would return, that alcohol would allow me to appear to be normal, to function. I was in the terminal stages and I was beginning to have serious health problems. . . .

Like what?

The beginnings of alcoholic neuropathy, losing sensation in my hands and feet. Slicing my feet on broken glass and not knowing it. Being unable to eat. Everything was just drinking, drinking, drinking.

I was living with my sister, who was trying to get me to stop drinking. I had a terrifying experience with DTs where I was up on the window ledge and she was coming at me trying to get me down. But I saw her approaching with an enormous box of cockroaches. There were roaches all over the floor, all over the bed, all over the walls. And I was up on the window ledge trying to get away from them. I was screaming and she was throwing them at me. When in fact, all she was doing was trying to reach for me to get me down off the window sill. When I snapped out of it she was still trying to reach for me. I didn't go through the window but I could have. She kept putting her hand on the bed and saying, "See, there's nothing here, there's nothing here." Suddenly I could see that there weren't any bugs. It was as if, the feeling was as if someone had just pulled all the bones out of my body, I don't know if you've ever had that feeling. I just went limp. She pulled me down and put me to bed.

But I continued going to all the quack doctors, trying to find the magic, not a way to stop drinking, but to be able to drink and not have these things happen, which, I don't know, I think is fairly classic. Not all of the doctors asked me about my drinking. Some would, and of course I would lie. I would say I have one or two, but I didn't say one or two *what*. By then it was vast amounts—bottles. I never had one or two glasses. I drank bottles every day, all day. I drank at work. I put booze in my coffee. I had little miniatures in my pockets and I lived in fear of running out. Finally, I could not get a job.

My friend Emmett finally said, "You need help. Will you go see a psychiatrist?" And I said, "Yes." The psychiatrist had an office in the East 50s and while I was sitting there waiting for her to come in, I noticed a lot of the books on her shelves had the word alcoholism in their titles. And so I made some smart-ass crack when Dr. [Ruth] Fox★ sat down. "Why are you so preoccupied with alcoholism?" It never dawned on me that that was the reason I was there. For some reason, I was able to tell her pretty much the truth to the best of my ability. I think it was because of my friend Emmett. His simple gesture, making the appointment with Dr. Fox, was the beginning of a very long journey back. I was being fairly arrogant and smart-alecky about it. At the end of the session she said, "Well, do you know what your problem is?" And I said, "No, *you* tell *me*, that's why I'm here." And she took out a prescription pad and wrote something on it and handed it to me and it said, "A.A." She said, "Will you go?" I said I'd think about it. Then she asked me if I'd heard of Antabuse and I said no and she explained that to me. She said, "Would you take that? Do you want to stop drinking?" Well, I didn't, of course. I just wanted to get out of there and have a drink. But I didn't want to say anything to get her mad, so I said yes and she said all right. Then she opened this big jar of Antabuse and took

---

★*Dr. Ruth Fox was famous for treating alcoholics. She also introduced Antabuse, a drug that makes one very ill when taken with alcohol, to the United States.*

some out. I said, "Well, I'll take one later." She said, "No, take one now." So she gave me the pill and I took it. And she, being no fool, made sure I swallowed it.

It was a morning appointment and I remember, though I wouldn't dream of being seen at A.A., I thought nothing of staggering in an elevator full of people in this East 50s apartment building, trying to get that pill up. Trying to gag and force it up. And I did that. But it was too late and I was stuck.

Then I decided with typical alcoholic logic I would immunize myself to Antabuse. I began my experiment. My sister, who knew about Antabuse, was doling them out daily. So I would take small increments of alcohol, get violently sick, have heart palpitations, act generally insane and have dreadful physical reactions while trying to build up an immunity to Antabuse. Finally, at her wits' end, Fox said, "Let's try LSD." And I said, "Well, what does that do?" She said, "It will help us get at the roots." I guess she was still concerned—there was that body of experts who are concerned with what *causes* alcoholism. Trying to ponder the imponderable. With all her knowledge, she was still doing that. Now, bear in mind that at that point in time, Bill Wilson* was also fiddling around with LSD. Nobody knew how dangerous it was. But here I am, already hallucinating and being given an hallucinogen. So I said, "All right, give it to me," thinking it would unravel those terrible problems that were happening every time I drank. I wanted to be able to drink. Well, it was terrifying. I think, if I'm not mistaken, I think Fox stopped experimenting with LSD after that experience. I mean, I was out of my mind. It was crazy. Finally I stopped my experiments with Antabuse and the drinking and gave up. Not drinking—Antabuse.

Meanwhile everyone in my life had left. My sister probably went off into an unfortunate first marriage because of my drinking. I mean, here she had observed as a small child her mother's deterioration, and now she was watching the madness in spades with me. I was full of denial—lying. How could I tell anyone the truth when I couldn't admit it to myself?

I went into public relations and I became a press agent. While you shouldn't be drunk and be a press agent, I was a very good press agent. My life was now utter, sheer desperation. I was drinking

*Bill Wilson was the co-founder of Alcoholics Anonymous.

around the clock, the hallucinations were increasing. I went on a lot of national publicity tours with stars. Marilyn Monroe was a client of our firm. I did not handle her, another woman in the office did. But after I got sober I realized that Marilyn was an alcoholic too and that there's probably no mystery to her death, she died a classic alcoholic death. All the other stuff was melodrama. What we're looking at was tragic, a terrible waste. She smelled. I smelled. The one time that I had any exposure to her, she said to me, "Now honey, when I ask you to get me a glass of water, don't bring me water, bring me vodka." And my thought was, "Oh boy, we're going to get along just great." Yet when she died, it didn't connect that the glasses of vodka were probably behind it.

I would go on these publicity tours. I would be running for planes I had just gotten off. I mean, I don't know how I did it. But I was working frantically to cover up so no one would guess my secret. I began to have seizures in the office. The only thing I would not drink was gin. I could not abide the smell, the taste, because that was what my mother drank and my mother was an alcoholic and I was damned if I was going to be an alcoholic.

One day I woke up and I usually had a bottle in the bed or next to the bed on the floor so I could have a drink in order to get up. I woke up and the bottle was empty so I broke the bottle and tried licking the glass.

Oh God.

It wasn't enough and I had to get to work. So I fell out of bed, threw myself onto the floor and pulled myself with my elbows across the floor to the closet where I kept, you know the old cloth shoe bags? Well, I didn't keep shoes in there, I kept bottles. My bedroom supply. I don't know where the shoes were. I had the shakes so badly I couldn't get the bottle uncorked, or by this time it was probably the cheap stuff, and I couldn't get the cap off. I was shaking and shaking, I had to have the drink, I had to get up, I had to go to work. I couldn't miss work. If you missed work, that meant you were an alcoholic and I was not going to be an alcoholic. I broke the neck of the bottle and I couldn't get it into my mouth, it kept missing and it lacerated my lips and went all over my face.

It was vodka because I believed it didn't smell. I got some down and it came right up. So then I went through that whole thing again. I got it down. I held my mouth shut and it came right up and out my nose. I did it again, held my mouth shut, my nose shut, and I forced it down and then I was able, finally, to get to my feet, go into the bathroom and perform the morning ritual of throwing up. I would wash my face, brush my teeth, get dressed and have a few more stiff belts, then put my little bottles in my coat pockets.

Crossing a street was a nightmare. With the miniatures in my pockets—I waited at the light and took a drink. I'd walk really close to the sides of the buildings. I had tremendous vertigo, fear of falling over. This is how I would get to work. I always had a bottle in my purse and had to walk regally so it wouldn't gurgle when I came in. Then I would just slip it into my desk and have it with my coffee all day long. And this is how I lived. Around the clock, every waking moment ingesting alcohol in one form or another.

I had no life, my friends were gone . . . those who suggested that drinking might be the problem, I just eliminated. I stopped going out because I couldn't stand having to watch how I drank or trying to control it and having only one so people wouldn't talk about alcoholism to me. I was showing them that I wasn't an alcoholic but my mind was always racing, *"When can I get the hell out of here and go home and have a real drink?"* And so I just stopped going out. And I remember thinking, this has got to stop. I was in that in-between— too sick to die, too sick to live—stage. So I had a little drink to annihilate the feeling. I'm not sure if it was that same day or a few days later, but apparently I collapsed in the bathroom at the office and they had to break the door down to get me out. They didn't know what was wrong with me. The way I reeked? They didn't guess what was wrong with me? Then I had a seizure and was sent to Bellevue. In those days, no hospital would admit you for alcoholism, we were too much trouble.

There was one hospital in New York that had five beds for alcoholics. No public or private hospitals wanted you. I went to Bellevue three times and was let right out. Another time was when I was back out on a window ledge. A neighbor across the way saw me and got me down and I know I was screaming. I was tied up. I didn't want to be seen. So I had anonymity too. Alcoholics are invisible. Even now you see alcoholics lying in doorways and people walk right by. We have no faces, we are truly anonymous, even within our own families. I knew all about anonymity. Erased myself for booze. And if I did remember things, then I would eradicate them with booze. And now I would wake up in strange places and sometimes my body would be racked with pain and I would look at the form in the bed and I wouldn't know what I had done. I felt so degraded, I couldn't even tell my sponsor.

Was Marty Mann* your sponsor from the beginning?

No, my first sponsor was a little, tough, street-wise woman who was assigned to me. She was a waitress in a coffee shop and had been a former Roller Derby queen. She was some tough cookie. She was my first sponsor and Marty became my sponsor when I moved to Connecticut. She was my second sponsor and remained my sponsor right up until she died.

All that information I had held in came out one night at a big open meeting here in Westport that we call "The Bakeoff," about 300 people attended it. It was a two-speaker meeting and as I walked in, one of the guys came up to me and said, "Oh good, you're here. Our speakers haven't shown up. Will you go on?" And I was completely unprepared. I stood up in front of all those people and I began to speak and all this *stuff* came out. The most dreadful, the worst secrets, all the things I had done, all the degradation and humiliation just flowed out. Afterwards, many people came up to me and put their arms around me and hugged me. I knew something remarkable had happened. . . . I had in some way been touched by something. The following Friday I was at my home group, and one of the men said during the discussion, "On Wednesday, I was at a meeting and someone in this room spoke. It was the most profound experience of my sobriety." He said, "It was a story so honestly told, it felt as though we all being touched by God's grace. I will never forget it as long as I live." I just started to cry with relief that I wasn't hallucinating. This man had felt whatever it was, too. It was one of the many thresholds, those awakenings that we all experience. In the beginning I wanted the big theatrical one like Bill's blinding white light, Marty Mann seeing red, the things you read about in the literature. I didn't have those. Looking back I can see the first in-

---

**Marty Mann was the first woman to recover in A.A. See her story on page 214.*

crement was in the moment the thought crossed my mind on the closet floor that *this has got to stop.*

The next time was some months later when I took a geographic cure to the coast, unauthorized, on the company credit cards, staying with people who neither drank nor smoked. I really thought if I went out there that I could get my life together. It was New York. It was my job. It was all these influences that were causing the problems. Once I got to California it would be all right. Of course it wasn't.

You know, people don't walk in California, they drive everywhere. I did the inevitable, I found a liquor store and walked to it and I got—I was just going to get a little vodka, for a little cocktail that I would have out in the bushes before I went into the house. But I wound up buying two quarts. I remember going into this bush next to the house. It was July and the sun was very intense. I held the bottle up—it was like this giant prism refracting magically in the intense light, liquid crystal, magic. I was really happy with anticipation of the magic, with belief that the magic would return. The next thing I remember, it was dark and I was face down under a car and a guy was kicking me in the side. I heard a voice say, "Is she dead?" and another one say, "Nah, she's just an alcoholic." And then I was dragged up into the grass.

I can remember years before fighting with my mother over a bottle. She'd hidden her booze in the garage and so had I. She had gotten what I thought was my bottle and I had gotten what she thought was her bottle and we fought like two cats in a bag over it. I can remember her saying to me that night, "You'll wind up in the gutter." And while it was a grassy, clean gutter, it was a gutter all right. Then I promptly vomited. I remember telling this at Lenox Hill, which is one of the oldest groups in New York, the Fifth Avenue group where all the dowager alcoholics went wearing their diamond collars and their minks and sables. A very regal woman came up to me afterwards and said, "Dahling, why did you say 'vomit'?" I thought for a moment and said, "Because that's what it was." I said, "What should I say?" and she said, "Upchuck." And I thought and said, "No, this wasn't upchuck, this was vomit. This was the bottom of hell I was lying face down in. It was all the rot from my insides. It was vomit all right." She just grinned and walked away. Anyway, I'm lying there and I thought simply two words, and they were, "Oh God." I knew in that moment that I was dying and I knew it

was taking too long. The plea, the forlorn cry was, "Just let me die."
You know. Just take me. And it was, I think, the beginning of the
next phase of my surrender.

The next day I woke up. I obviously didn't die. I was covered
with filth, still in my clothes, in the bed. Apparently there was a
mad chase all over the neighborhood while they tried to get me back
in the house. I had no memory of that, but you know, somebody
will tell you what you did if you wait around long enough. The best
defense is an offense. *I'm going back to New York, it's all California,
it's all these people.* I was just horrible to everyone. They brought me
a car, and I couldn't even write my name on the rental slip. Meanwhile, I had changed into a dress; I hadn't bathed or showered and
Hertz gave me the car anyway. I guess out there, even then, they
were used to seeing strange sights. But instead of going to the airport,
I drove across the valley and I was going seven miles an hour, my
right leg snapping up in the air above the accelerator, hanging onto
the wheel and I felt as though a piano wire was being drawn around
my midsection. Shaking and sweating, I went to see this woman
and I'm not even quite sure how I met her. I did something I'd never
in my life done before. I told her my story. She broke her anonymity
and asked if I wanted help and in that moment I did.

I got back to New York and apparently got back into my apartment
and started drinking again. When I came to I didn't know whether
it was day or night, or what month it was, or when I'd last been to
work. I was really frightened. Desperately, I dialed "0" and the
operator connected me with A.A. The office had an answering machine and I left my name and number. I got dressed, or I thought I
got dressed and I went down onto the street and hailed a cab to take
me to a meeting. What I had never seen in the sixteen years that I
lived and drank in that neighborhood was that one of the oldest
meetings in Manhattan met probably twenty-nine steps from my
apartment door. They had signs out in front. I never saw them. I
had no idea where A.A. was. So the cab driver took me to the Bowery
Mission, which is for men but they were nice to me. I remember
them bringing me in and handing me a cup of coffee and a donut
and I don't remember anything else.

The next morning I was awakened by a woman with a Bronx
accent. She was returning my call from the night before and she said,
"Do you want help?" and I said,"Yes." She said, "Do you have a
bottle?" And I said, "Yes." There was a bottle on the bureau. I was

sitting on the floor with the phone on my lap. She said, "Is the cork in the bottle?" And I said, "No," and she said, "Well, put it in the bottle." And I said, "I can't." And she said "Why not?" and I said, "Because if I touch the bottle, I'll take a drink." She said, "In that case, don't put the cork in the bottle. If someone comes, will you let them in?" I said, "Yes," I said I would try and go unlock the door. She said, "I'll hold on while you go do that." I had to crawl to the door and unlock it and then I crawled back to the phone. She said "I'll call you back and let you know when someone's coming." She tried that whole day, it was October 15, a Saturday, and she couldn't get anybody. No one came. She called me every ten minutes and talked to me, she talked me down. At one point I remember I was lying on the carpet, terrified that I was going to fall over the edge, just screaming and hanging on for dear life. I'd look at that bottle and I'd look at the phone and the phone would ring. I kept hoping someone would come and no one came. Finally she said, "Do you think you can get to a meeting?" I said I would try, so she gave me the address. It was the old Carlyle group and they met in a church on 59th Street.

I'll never forget facing those doors, it had taken me forever to get to them. I mean, I had no money. I think I had used my last bit of cash going down to the Bowery Mission. I was facing those doors, those Gothic doors, and thinking, "How will I ever do this? How will I ever cross this street? How will I ever get in there?" It took every ounce of energy to propel myself through the doors. I got in and there was this little old guy setting up chairs. I said, "Where is everybody?" I thought it would be full of people. He said, "Oh, they're not here yet. Are you here for a meeting?" And I remember thinking, "Gee, I wonder how he knows?" Bear in mind I was missing two front teeth and had a black eye and was probably 180 pounds of pure alcoholic bloat. I have no idea how I lost my teeth, got the black eye—falling I think. Looking for booze. I lived alone, I hid the booze. I'd tear the apartment apart looking for it. If you saw it in a movie, you'd say, "Oh, *please*, too melodramatic." I could barely stand up and I said, "Well, I'll go for a walk and come back." And he said, "No, no, you sit down." He wasn't even in the program. So I sat down; I don't remember anything about the meeting. What I do remember was the health in the room, I felt safe. And being shocked by the laughter and the humor and the warmth. People walked me home and picked me up the next day. I was carried, literally, in relays, to meetings. I had no idea what everybody was talking about for the longest time.

I think the final part of recovery, the awakening, was one night at my home group, which was the Sutton group, because I lived off Sutton Place. I always sat in the back of the room. The only job I was capable of performing was, they wouldn't let me pick up the ashtrays after the meeting because I spilled them, but they let me put them down on the chairs. That was my job. So I had to get there early because it took me a long time to get around the room with the ashtrays. I developed a discipline that I have to this day—I'm always at least a half an hour early to a meeting. Anyhow, I somehow got caught putting ashtrays up front and I turned around to go to the back of the room, and it was full, so I had to sit there up front. I was looking at the speaker, who was a woman whom I've never seen again. Maybe if she reads your book and she'll recognize this, and she'll know who she is and know I thank her. She saved my life. I now know I was ready to go back out and drink.

I sat there looking at that woman, she looked so nice. In those days, they always told you to try and look your best. When you went on speaking dates, you dressed for it—stockings, shoes, skirt. Now I go in sneakers and jeans like everybody else. Her nails were almond-shaped and perfect. She had on very understated but nice gold jewelry. Her hair was lovely, and I thought, "*You* have never been where I've been. *You* have never felt what I've felt or known what I've known." The rage was unbelievable. Then I noticed as she went to light a cigarette that her hand was trembling. I think this was when the real miracle happened for me. I thought, "My god, she's nervous." And in that moment I became interested in another human being. I think that's when my recovery began. I listened to her as I've never listened to anyone as she told her story—it was far more graphic, far more horrible than anything I had known. She had wound up in the Bowery sucking booze off a filthy washrag that was clogging up a flophouse sink, where she had repaired with some guy in order to get a drink. And she had cut her own throat in a blackout and luckily was found. She had gone to hell and back again. In that moment I understood what I had heard at every meeting back in the beginning, which I don't hear so much anymore, which was try to identify with the feelings, not the events. Even with all this dreadful stuff, she had gone farther and lower than I had gone— there was a single word that she uttered, and it was *loneliness*. It was like the fog lifting from my mind. I knew she had been where I had been and felt what I had felt. I listened to that story and I thought, "My god, if she could come back and recover from that, then maybe, just maybe, I could do it too." I have never been able to forget any of that. It was drilled into me early on that I must keep those memories green. I know people in my family who are not in the program will say, "Do you still go to those meetings that you used to go to?" And I say yes. They ask, "Well, how often do you go?" I say, "At least five times a week." "Five times a week?" they scream, and I say, "Yes," and they say, "Well, why?" and I say, "What if no sober people had been there the night I had fallen through the door?"

When I speak I always make a point of saying, "You do not have to do what I did. I don't know why I lived through it, because most people don't, when they go into the terminal stages." I say, "I'm only telling you this so you'll know what's there if you keep going and you probably won't live through it. There are three things an alcoholic has to look forward to, three choices we can make. One is madness, two—the morgue with a tag around our toe, or sobriety. It's that simple. When I came into the program people died in the meetings from alcoholic withdrawal. We understood very clearly that this was a life or death matter. This wasn't your dog peed on your Oriental carpet. This is life or death business."

August 1990

Denise Mindham

Born Denise Real in Santa Cruz, California, in 1958, to a mother who is a Jehovah's Witness, and an alcoholic father, at sixteen she ran away from home and became a prostitute. About her father she said, "He was a plasterer, a plastered plasterer, and we were always broke." About her mother, "She rejected me because I refused to become a Jehovah's Witness. The relationship is dead. I need to grieve it. And I would have been such a good daughter. No one believes that my mother did this to me." At age thirty-two she uses the affirmations in Women for Sobriety to give herself the love she was never given as a child. She is five feet four and slim with short blonde hair. She lives in Juneau, Alaska, with her husband, Michael, and works for a major airline. A certified moderator for Women for Sobriety, she works in her spare time as a United Way campaign manager. She has been sober since 1987.

At my first A.A. meeting I said, "Hi, my name is Denise. I'm an alcoholic and I'm never going to drink again." They told me I couldn't say that, that I didn't *know* that. Finally, for once in my life, I'd taken control and decided I was going to be the dictator of my life and they said I mustn't do that. I'd finally set one goal in my life, for sobriety, and they were saying I couldn't do it.

I'm very strong-willed. I'm more than just a survivor, I'm a thriver. I was a very good alcoholic. No matter what I set my mind to do, I'm very good at it. I resented it terribly when they told me that I couldn't say I would never drink again. I said, "There is nothing in my life that could ever be so bad as to make me take another drink, or smoke another joint, or snort another line, or take another pill." Now, finally, I have my own life. For twenty-nine years it was everybody's life but mine. I'd never made an attempt before at sobriety. I wasn't one of those who tried, relapsed, tried, relapsed. I've only tried to get sober one time, and I did it.

Did you go back to A.A.?

I went to a couple of meetings. I guess you have to go back to the beginning to understand why I didn't like it.

My mother's a Jehovah's Witness. I'm the youngest of three girls. My father's an alcoholic. My mother became a Jehovah's Witness when I was about five years old. Her three daughters were forced into her religion by her, which is something I believe she turned to because of my father's drinking. It worked out well for both of them because his alcoholism enabled her to be a Jehovah's Witness and her religion enabled him to be an alcoholic. They fed each other's diseases.

Do you think the intensity of your mother's religion made it difficult for you to be receptive to A.A.?

Definitely. I was forced into her religion. To this day my mother doesn't claim me as her daughter. I'm dead in her eyes because according to her, I know the truth and I'm not doing anything about it. I walked away from her religion. The only way I can get acceptance and love from my mother . . . this is really hard (crying), it hurts . . . is to be a part of that religion. That's something I'm still trying to deal with. It's a relationship that I really needed. It's a conditional love thing and it's total bullshit. There's nothing I can do about it; it's just something I have to accept. It's her disease. I've accepted mine. It's very frustrating. I try to say that I'm over it, and that I understand it, and that I'm not going to be hurt by it any more. But those are just words because I *am* hurt by it.

It's frustrating because when *I* started changing my family wouldn't. There still wasn't going to be any love there. I've had a double whammy from my mother. Being the youngest of three girls, turning off to this religion completely, and finally coming out and being able to admit, "Look, I don't believe this shit, Ma, and you shouldn't either. But that's your choice. I'm not going to."

When I was sixteen I ran away to Alaska and didn't contact anybody for a long, long time. Both of my sisters resent that. They had to stay there and I got to leave. Especially my oldest sister. She had to stay with my alcoholic father. I decided not to have anything to do with anybody. It's what I had to do to live. I feel the choices that I made were the right ones at the time. I didn't feel like I had anything else to do but run away. When my sisters turned eighteen, they got married and moved out of the house. All of a sudden there I was, fifteen years old, stuck in a house with a woman I hated, and a drunken asshole.

When did you start drinking?

There was always beer around. That was my father's drink of choice. I think I started drinking heavily when I was about fourteen. When I was in ninth grade I started hanging out with the kids at school drinking Boone's Farm apple wine. When I was fifteen, I started smoking marijuana. I moved in with my sister and started drinking hard liquor and doing acid. Anything I could get my hands on. I just went wild, totally wild.

I got into some trouble with the police for siphoning gas, of all things. Plus, I hadn't been going to school. I had to choose between going back to school, juvenile hall, or going to something in San Jose, California, called Job Service. I wasn't doing well in school and I certainly didn't want to go back to living with my parents. I didn't want to go to jail, to juvenile hall, so I said I'd go to this Job Service thing.

I was there for about a month. While I was there I met a girl who said, "You know, I can teach you how to make some extra money." She introduced me to a pimp. I didn't know a thing about prostitution, not a thing. I was very promiscuous. I didn't even have to know your name to go to bed with you. I believe this was part of the disease, the low self-esteem I got from my family. I didn't place any value on myself. I found that by offering myself sexually I was getting accepted.

I turned a few tricks for a guy in San Jose and he kept the money because I really didn't know what was going on. He sold me to a black guy from Fairbanks, a teamster and a pimp. His name was Leon Avery and he was quite a bit older than me. I was sixteen and he was in his thirties. Leon Avery bought me for a thousand dollars. He got me a fake ID and bought me a ring. We went to Reno and he married me there. He purchased some cocaine and took me and the cocaine up to Fairbanks.

Now, this guy's under the impression that he's buying a hooker. But I had never been turned out, taught how to be a prostitute, to get the money up front. When I was working for the guy in San Jose, I would just walk by and he'd find customers. He'd say, "This is the girl. Do you want her?" And I'd just go with them. So when Leon Avery gets me up to Fairbanks, he finds out that he's got a girl who doesn't know a thing about prostitution.

I stayed with him for quite a while. He was physically abusive. I went to bed with guys who were supposed to pay me and of course I didn't do it right and didn't get the money. They'd just sleep with me for free and he'd beat me severely for that. It was a real nightmare. He had given me an identity of Elizabeth Moore, and when he married me I became Elizabeth Avery

I was there almost a year, and finally I ran away from him. He kept trying to come back and kill me. At one point he came to a restaurant and took me out at gunpoint. He had me in his car. I was in the passenger side and he was in the driver's side. I put my foot on the gas pedal and crashed the car to give me time to get out. A truck full of teenagers coming by saw what happened and took me in.

I took him to court and got a restraining order against him. He ended up in jail for robbing a clothing store and I haven't seen him since. A couple of times I'd think I'd seen him and I'd freak out because he was trying to kill me. The whole time I was with him I was drinking and doing drugs. It's a big grey area for me. I never did get properly turned out.

I would live with any man who'd have me because I couldn't take care of myself. I worked at a dirty bookstore for a while, still under the alias of Elizabeth Avery. Otherwise I was underage to be doing anything.

We had what they called after-hours, party houses. I was living with a girlfriend and her boyfriend. They had an after-hours down in the basement of our home. I met a man there, a pimp, and his name was Sammy Dane. I was, you know, *please take me with you,* a very needy type of person, very dependent on drugs and men. Drugs, men, and sex were my addictions. Sammy Dane did take me in and he turned me out properly. I worked for him for about four years. This was during the construction of the oil pipeline and I made a lot of money. It was nothing to go out and make two thousand dollars a night on Two Street in Fairbanks. My spot there was the Polaris Lounge. I also worked out of a whorehouse called Ruthie's. Ruthie's closed down a couple of years ago. They put her out of business when the Chief of Police up in Fairbanks got in trouble for buying a Mercedes for his wife from her. Fairbanks is a real Peyton Place. It lives up to its reputation. They're trying to get the place cleaned up, but of course it's not easy to do now that Fairbanks is out of money, now that the pipeline jobs are gone.

I stayed with Sammy Dane for quite a while. He was heavy into dealing coke and I was into *doing* coke. My drink of choice was straight shots of Crown Royal, coke backed. I don't know how I could consume as much as I did in the course of an evening without dying of alcohol poisoning. Even now it amazes me how much I could drink.

Did you want to get out of the life?

Sometimes I did and sometimes I didn't. It was something I was very comfortable with. It was something I was very good at. I truly believed I was in love with Sammy Dane. He had other women, but I was his main lady, and I was in love with him. I'd ask him to marry me. I wanted to have his baby.

I had gotten hooked on cocaine. I was freebasing, I was shooting cocaine. It got to where my addiction was too much for him and I started fucking up. Not getting the money up front.

Did you need to be high to have sex?

No, sex was another addiction. I was co-addicted. I decided to leave him. I went down to California and then I went to Las Vegas for a while. I was terribly afraid of working on the streets in Las Vegas because I was afraid of going to jail. It was easy in Fairbanks where all the cops knew me. They weren't going to bust you unless you were stealing, unless you were breaking the law.

I called Sammy Dane up in Fairbanks and said I needed a ticket back to Fairbanks. When I got up there I told him that I didn't want to be in the life anymore. But I was still turning tricks off and on with people I knew. Instead of going back on the street full-time, I had a sugar daddy. I danced at a club, which was kind of the next step away from prostitution. When you're dancing you're either going into prostitution or coming out of it. I danced with a girlfriend at a place called the Goodtimers Club. I was just kind of going through the motions of life, I wasn't really living. I still had a very bad cocaine habit. I was still shooting cocaine and drinking really heavily. It was very convenient to work in a bar, especially in a bar where you're dancing. Guys buy you drinks. Everything was just right for my survival.

Finally, I didn't want to do it anymore. I had moved into the Northwood building downtown. I was still drinking heavily, smoking a lot of weed, cocaine, whatever I could get my hands on. But I quit dancing and got a job driving a school bus. Next stop, right? I wouldn't drink or snort coke before I drove the bus, but as soon as the run was over and the last child got off, I'd light up a joint. I'd go directly from the bus barn to the bar. Between that job and my sugar daddy it was enough to get by.

And then I met my husband. He worked as a maintenance person in the building where I lived. We shot pool together. He started adamantly pursuing me. At first I wasn't too interested. I'd sleep with him, but after that I really didn't want to see him again. He was persistent and we started a relationship. I moved in with him. It started out like a real relationship, as real as a dysfunctional relationship can get. We were both drinking heavily and smoking a lot of marijuana. He didn't do that much coke because he couldn't afford it, but I could.

He didn't want me turning any tricks. He had made plans to go down to Denver to go to diesel mechanic school and he wanted me to go with him. He left and I joined him there, about a month afterwards. We got married in 1983.

We finally got enough money together to move back to Fairbanks. We wanted to move back to Alaska because that way he didn't have to pay back all of his student loans. We weren't making enough money in California, anyway. So we moved back to Fairbanks and

I went to work for a travel agency. I was still drinking real heavy. He was working at the Northwood building again as the assistant manager and maintenance foreman. It's a huge complex of apartments and covers a whole city block in Fairbanks. I worked for a travel agency for a month and they went out of business, so I went to work for another travel agency. I was having these two–or–three martini-type lunches. Even though my sales were real good the managers were saying, "You've got a problem with alcohol." I told my husband that I wanted to go back to school. I was getting in trouble at my job. I was trying to control my drinking. The whole time, when we were in Denver, and sometimes in Fairbanks, he'd say, "Let's go on the wagon for a month." I'd say, "Yeah, okay, no problem," and I'd do it just to keep him off my back. But I knew the minute the thirty days was up I was going to get shit-faced. When we were on the wagon we wouldn't drink but we'd smoke marijuana. I'd take pills—Excedrin PM, Valiums, anything I could get my hands on. We'd be in the bars downtown at night. I'd get drunk and we'd get in fights with each other and with other people. It was quite a life.

I was so proud of myself in Fairbanks because I thought I was a normal person. I wasn't on the streets anymore. I had a real job, and when I didn't, I went to the community college. I was still drinking real heavy. And if somebody offered cocaine, I'd snort it. But I wasn't *shooting* cocaine anymore.

I took a job about three and a half years ago working with a major airline in Alaska. It's a company based in Seattle that does cruise ship tours. I went to work for them for a season as a receptionist. One weekend my girlfriend and I went to Mount McKinley, to Denali Park. They gave us a free room and everything, and we both got shit-faced. I did all sorts of horrible things. I told them I was the manager of the company. I went back to work Monday morning. My boss didn't know I had a drinking problem. She didn't know anything about alcoholism. She said, "I can't believe this. I don't know what to do. They want me to *fire* you." I don't remember half of what she was talking about because I was totally blacked out. Finally I said, "Look, Nancy, I've really got a problem. I think I'm an alcoholic." So she said, "Well, we're going to have to do something for you." She, my husband, and I, we all got together. He was really concerned. He was afraid I would leave him if he said he wanted me to stop drinking, which is really unusual. Statistically, it's only one in ten men who stay with women alcoholics.

Are you still married?

Yeah, you bet. It'll be eight years in June.

We checked into going into treatment centers but we couldn't afford it. They wanted eight thousand dollars to go into a twenty-one day program. Finally we found an outpatient program. It was a state funded outpatient program that I could go to and our insurance would pay for eighty percent of it. I had to go to a detox center for five days to qualify for it. My boss at work was so understanding and so helpful. She told me to take a week off and told everybody I had the flu. I was very lucky there. I did the detox thing, which was really scary.

When I got out of the outpatient program I went to my first A.A. meeting, the one where I was told that you can't say you'll never drink again because you don't know that. It was very hard for me because at this Alcoholics Anonymous meeting there were a lot of men who used to be my tricks. A lot of the women there knew who I was, and knew I used to be on the streets, and knew that I used to sleep with their husbands. It was impossible for me to recover in that setting.

It's hard to put your past behind you when it's sitting in front of you. I couldn't stand up in front of these people and tell my story when it involved half the men in the room. (Crying.) I couldn't say I got so shit-faced, not only did I go to bed with one of those guys, but he was so drunk that I ripped half his money off and he never knew it. This is the type of thing they talk about there. I certainly wasn't going to get up and tell them that. I couldn't tell about the times when I got so fucked up it took me thirty minutes to shoot my arm up. Or about the time one night that I got so drunk that I decided to turn three tricks at one time. They're going to sit there and listen to that? No. I don't think so.

I was trying to overcome my alcoholism. I had already gotten past that other life. I didn't want to go back into that. I didn't want to open that back up. (Crying.)

It was very strange that we would even go back to Fairbanks

considering my history there. My husband asked, "Is this going to
be a problem for you?" and I said, "No, it's not." It wasn't a problem
even though occasionally I would run into Sammy Dane, the pimp
I was with for so many years. He'd say, "When you coming home?"
He was always saying that, you know, "When you coming home?"
I'd say, "I *am* home, just leave me alone." I guess they're all still
dysfunctional and on the streets up there.

I had a dream the other night about Suzy, one of my stable sisters.
I dreamt that we were going to a Women for Sobriety meeting and
we had gotten stoned. I still have these really weird dreams. I'm still
feeling guilty.

*How did you get in touch with Women for Sobriety? How did you hear
about it?*

When I left the A.A. meeting I went to a bookstore. I was very
upset that things had gone the way they had because I had expected
to go in there and have everybody say, "Yeah. All right. You're
changing your life!" The response that I got was you can't do it that
way. What you want, you can't have. I had a very good counselor
though, he was very supportive. I could tell him my whole story
and he didn't judge me. He was very nice. (Crying.) I had a lot of
sexual hang-ups. I learned about sex by reading books that my dad
would leave lying around, the *Debbie Does Dallas* porno-type thing.
My image of sex was so twisted and warped. It was so easy for me
to get into *the life* because that's what I thought it was supposed to
be. I thought perverse sex was natural. He made a point, he said,
"Did you ever think that maybe your dad left those books out for
you to read on purpose?" It was something I hadn't really thought
about, and something I still wonder about. When you start talking
to women alcoholics, the number of women that were sexually
abused as children is startling. I'm one of them.

My counselor worked in a bookstore and he'd always said, "The
key to your recovery is going to be education." I believe that so
much now, because I really didn't know anything about the disease,
even though I'd had so much contact with it. Even though I was an
adult child of an alcoholic, I knew nothing about it. I read all kinds

of books. I got two of Jean Kirkpatrick's★ books, and I read them and I was very excited about Women for Sobriety. In Fairbanks there wasn't anything but Alcoholics Anonymous. There wasn't a Women for Sobriety group.

Six months into my recovery we moved to Juneau. I wrote to Women for Sobriety to see if there was a group around here. I wanted to get more information. They said, "There's not a group, but would you like to start one?" I said, "No, I'm not ready for that." So I practiced the program on my own. I was the only person in my group for two years.

Did you read the affirmations in the morning?

Yes. I had cards all over, little affirmations here and there. I got up in the morning and did meditation. I was feeling very good. I changed my life completely. I had put on quite a bit of weight. My weight had gone up to about 185 pounds. I joined a diet center and lost all that weight. I quit smoking, quit drinking, quit drugging, and quit eating. I started exercising regularly and became physically and mentally healthy. It took two years to do all of this recovery. It was a hard decision to make, but I did it.

In the beginning of April I said, "This is the time for me to start a group for Women for Sobriety." I was tired of being the only person in my group. (Laughs.) I felt like there was something missing in my life. I thought, "Maybe what I need is to try religion again." I started a Women for Sobriety group and threw myself into it, going and talking to women about W.F.S.

The initial response from the woman would be great and then I wouldn't see her again. It was very frustrating.

How did you find women?

Well, the first thing I did was, I got a phone line put in just for Women for Sobriety. I set up a little back office in a back bedroom that I didn't use. It was strictly a Women for Sobriety line because

---

★ *Jean Kirkpatrick founded Women for Sobriety, an alternative to A.A. See her story on page 159.*

I wanted to do it right. I wanted it separate from my other things. I made up about two hundred flyers and put them all around town. I took information to all the recovery centers here in town. I sent it to all the different counselors and I got in touch with the Alaska Council on Alcoholism and Drug Abuse. I just started knocking on doors and putting posters up.

I began getting calls from people that were interested. I met a woman named Kathryn King. She and I are the only two real members you can count on always being there. A lot of times we'll have a meeting and we'll be the only ones that show up.

At one point I got a call from a woman who said she thought she had a drinking problem but she didn't want to go to A.A. because it was full of lesbians and hookers. Well lady, if you only knew. I tried to tell her, "Alcoholism doesn't discriminate." If she'd known I'd worked the pipeline... (laughs). Everyone thinks I'm this nice little housewife who used to drink too much.

That need I had felt for something religious was working for me in W.F.S. I found that I was growing.

The affirmations really do help?

Yes. It's absolutely true what's said about us: as long as you have one negative thought, you can't have anything positive. I still have my days when I have trouble, and I have to sit down and think about how far I've come. I've been sober for three years. It was three years on the first of July.

And it's all been through Women for Sobriety?

Yes. The whole program is about self-esteem, self-worth. I had none of that. I didn't give a shit about myself. I didn't care what happened to me. I didn't even know I was supposed to have self-esteem. I didn't know I was supposed to care about myself. I knew nothing about love. I was in love with men I'd just slept with. After fifteen minutes I'd say, "I love you." My relationship with my husband now is so good. My biggest and hardest step was learning to love myself.

That's what the program teaches, that I *am* worthy of love, that

I *am* beautiful. It's so nice to have that. Now I can do things for myself. I'm in control of my life.

Last year I went to a family reunion and I was talking to people down there, telling them I'm an alcoholic. The same people who were telling me I needed help were turning around and saying, "No, you're not an alcoholic. No, you couldn't be." Is this real? Am I on the right planet? It was a very rude awakening to go down there with this new life, and this wonderful husband whom I love—to go down there and find out that nothing ever changes. Nobody's changed but me and I can't change any of them. That was very hard to take.

It was an especially rotten blow to find out that no matter how much I changed, my mom still wasn't going to love me. There is only one thing I can do to get her love and that's become a Jehovah's Witness. That's truly what it boils down to with her.

Are you ever tempted to?

Are you kidding? Do you know what those people are like? As far as a religion goes, or a belief like that, I don't have any and I don't feel like I need any. It doesn't really matter to me how this goddamned earth got here. What matters to me is my life on this earth and what I do with it. The Women for Sobriety philosophy is "Forget the past." I'd love to, but I use it as a learning tool. I don't forget it; I just act as though it never happened. If it weren't for that past, I wouldn't be who I am now. It's what's made me so strong.

You know what I dread most? That my family will accuse me of deserting them.

September 1990

Alicia

Five feet two and slim with long black hair and huge brown eyes, she uses her hands to emphasize words and feelings. She sits up perfectly straight while talking, gesturing and carefully selecting what she is going to say next. She is thirty-eight years old. Unfortunately for the Elm Street Center, the detoxification unit where she works as a counselor, she is leaving her job in Massachusetts and moving to Florida. Her patients truly love her. Alicia has difficulty keeping a "professional distance" from her work. She admits freely that she takes her work home, that her patients are also her friends and are often on her mind. "I hope the center will replace me with another Hispanic woman," she remarked; "almost all of our patients are Hispanics." She has three daughters. She is separated from her husband, who is still using drugs. She has been sober since 1987.

There was sexual abuse in my mother's background. So my mother put that fear in us. I stayed married to my husband for twenty-one years with his drug abuse of heroin for the fear that if I met someone, how can I trust that someone with my daughter? So fear kept me in that marriage, in that dysfunctional marriage. Along with that, my mother put the insecurities. I thought that by marrying my husband, it would be a way out. Instead, it was a hole deeper than the hole I came out of because my husband kept those insecurities and added some more. So self-esteem was not there. The insecurities were humongous that I had to break as years went by.

I didn't go to work. "If you do go to work, you're not going to be able to find anything. Okay? So you do better staying home with the three kids. *"If you go out, and if you leave me, who do you really think is going to want you? I mean, come on. Look at yourself in the mirror."* Every time I looked at myself I heard my husband's voice behind me, "Look at yourself in the mirror." It didn't do much for me. It just brang me further, further down.

I went to a psychiatrist and was diagnosed a manic–depressive and he gave me pills that I took whenever I felt depressed. The depression lasted from morning to night. And the constant crying without knowing what I'm crying for. I was sitting in self-pity for myself of, *"I'm in this hole and there's no way out. I see no way out."* I couldn't even visualize a way out. So I kept on those pills.

What kind of pills?

They were Valiums. My mother had a nervous breakdown which she never came back from. My father did not drink. My mother did. My mother stopped her drinking when she got a bleeding ulcer. But when I was young she would be in the street, pollutedly drunk, men would be abusing her. She had taken the daughter role. Well, I took the mother role. *"Get upstairs, you're embarrassing me. Here's some black coffee. Let her sleep, Dad, let her sleep off the drunkenness."* And then pray, as I'm laying down goin' to sleep, that she doesn't do it again the next day.

After a while I started getting into her medicine cabinet because my mother used to take Valium for nerves. Every time I had a problem, that pill would take me away. Mentally.

So you started pills at a young age?

Yeah. I started pills at, I would say, age seventeen. I would take whatever was out there in the market. 'Cause I come from a poverty area. I come from the Lower East Side in Manhattan where if you have an apartment, be grateful. There were not too many people who were gung ho, full of having goals and wanting to succeed in life. They felt they'd succeeded all they're going to succeed. A lot of the Hispanic people feel that way.

So what do you think the answer is? As a counselor, when you're with a patient who doesn't see a way out, what do you say?

I give them hope. By example. By me. And I do that in all of my meetings. There was one time that I used to be afraid to talk about my life. Years of therapy took me out of that. There was one point in life that I hated my mother tremendously for the things that she'd done to me, for the insecurities that she'd put in me. Through therapy, I overcame that. I tell that story to my patients. I'm not saying that the majority of the people start drugging at an early age. Some start experimenting and take the experiments further, until it's not an experiment anymore, it's a way of life. Then some do it to escape from their childhood, to erase the pain that they went through. I'm one of the statistics that did it to erase most of my childhood. And it became a way of life to me. Whenever I was in a situation I couldn't get out of, I'd take some pills. Drink. And not be able to think about it. But yet when you get up the next morning, those problems are still there, so you take some more pills and you drink and hope that they will go away by themselves. That eventually maybe someone can find a solution for you without you having to do the legwork for it. That was me.

What I do is I bring my story across to my patients. When I bring my story across, it's not a typical childhood life growing up. It's gruesome. When I tell them everything I've been through and they see where I am now—with that I am giving them hope that there is a better tomorrow. But you have to work at it. You have to believe in something.

I didn't know about A.A. I didn't know about N.A. I was trying to get my life together plus get my husband's life together. It was one addict helping another. I got my help through finding a Higher Power, through church, through religion, through finding a one-on-one relationship with the Lord. Now I go through changes in life but I don't want to go back to drugs. Nothing can be so bad as where I was.

I fear relapsing every day in my life. I think a lot of recovering addicts fear relapsing. I tell them what I carry with me is the four years I've had clean. I carry the monkey on my back of how I relapsed and where it took me. I see where I am right now. I don't want to go back. And I remember it vividly, like I put it on tape, and I play it back in my mind. And that helps me.

I do an inventory and I tell patients, "Work your program, work your twelve steps. Once you start getting your self-esteem back a little bit, then do a personal inventory—where you was, where you're at now, and where you would like to be. List the goals that you want to achieve. And as you get there, check them off. It's like going to a store. You know what's in your cabinet now and you know what's missing. Okay, you write down a list and you go into the store and you say, Well, I've got sugar in the house, but I don't have rice. So you put that in and you check it off." Your life is like that. You check off things that you've done, leaving things that you want to do for another day."

The thing that's rewarding to me is having seen these people being clean. Having seen these people being able to hold a *job*. Having seen these people happy because they got a *car*. The most little, insignificant thing that they didn't have when they were drugging or when they were on booze, that they've achieved now. That to me is worth more than the paycheck that they give me.

My kids have hoed a hard row and they've successfully done it, so that's a plus. This one, my youngest, I've sheltered her a lot. (Points to her daughter.) The other two, no. The other two grew up with guns in the house, syringes, Methadone bottles. You name it, they found it.

How do you feel about taking heroin addicts and giving them Methadone? Do you think it's an addiction in place of heroin or do you think it helps?

It helps short-term. I think what they do that's wrong is when they take a heroin addict and put him as an outpatient and give him too much Methadone. A certain amount of milligrams to stabilize him, fine, but they're giving him a certain amount over. You're not helping that person because he's not getting the proper counselling. If you're going to put a person on Methadone—motivate that person to some day be drug-free.

Isn't Methadone more addictive than heroin?

Yes. It affects the calcium in your bones, it's worse than heroin. My philosophy? People should kick it cold turkey. Not that many

people can do it. There's some that can do it. But the fear of feeling
pain because they've been on heroin for so long is hard. Heroin has
taken away their thinking, has taken away every little pain that they
feel. These people don't know what it is to feel a minor cramp because
they've been on heroin so long. Heroin has shut down everything.
All their feelings, their pain, whatever little *pinch* that they'd been
able to feel.

*Heroin, is it worse than alcohol? The withdrawal, is it worse than
tranquilizers?*

   Tranquilizers are the most hardest withdrawal there is. It's worse
than heroin. Heroin, you'll have the shivers, you'll have the sweats,
you'll have the cramping. With tranquilizers, you can go into serious
convulsions, epileptic seizures. If you've been on tranquilizers that
long a time—I think the way the clinic does that, twenty-eight days
isn't enough. Just like being on Methadone for twenty-eight days. I
explain to people how it's going to take quite some time before your
normal physical aspects come back. Sleeping will be up and down
because it's going to take some time for your body to heal. I say,
"Don't think that when you go home that you're going to be able
to sleep a full eight hours, that you're not going to feel any discom-
fort. You still will feel some, but not enough to run back and go
get some more dope. Or not enough to go on something else to
relieve the pain, because you're only starting the whole nightmare
all over again." I think what they need after that is a healthy support
group. It's going to take some time for them to get back into society,
for them to get back to a normal way of living. They had messed
up their normal way of living. Their way of living is getting up,
then they have to go out and cop and use. Then they can feel like
me and you. And the next day and the next day and the next day,
until you're feeding that habit that's getting bigger and bigger. Okay?
So for them to come back to getting up in the morning, having a
cup of coffee or a cigarette, or a cup of coffee and a donut—it's going
to take them quite some time. Because their way of living has been
turned upside down.

Recovery goes beyond just putting down the drink. Do you agree?

   Yes. All new doors are opening. But the end is that people who
are recovering have successfully made it back into society's way of

living. They've successfully made it back into the way they want it to be. That in itself is a big achievement for all these people. They should be commended because the worst is over. They've got their life back in their control to do whatever they choose to do with it. For that they should be commended.

There's many kinds of addiction. There's women who are addicted to men, there's women who are addicted to eating habits. If you look at it, the alcohol addiction and the drug addiction is not any worse than being addicted to a man, that you need a man by your side, that you can't function without one. You know you're full, you ate already, but you've got a compulsion of wanting to eat some more. Or a compulsion for gambling. But the main thing is, if you're able to overcome that, that in itself is an achievement. That you were able to take your life and be in control of it again.

I look at my children who have been through *hell* when their father was a heroin addict. My kids, before syringes were even out, knew what an eyedropper was, knew how he made it, have held guns in their hands, okay? I've got a daughter that's twenty-three years old who went through college. I've got another daughter that's twenty that's been accepted to Fort Lauderdale College and is going to be a fashion designer. I've got a thirteen-year-old who, I got group therapy for her for the fear that her father might have AIDS. It scared her for the fear that maybe I might have it. But we have a support group, me and my children. We have each other. No matter what we go through, we do it together and we hold onto each other. And that to me is a blessing, that my kids are able to overcome what they overcame and have made it. They need a gold medal. Because *me* as a child, raised in the era that I was raised in, in the sixties, if I would have had to see syringes, put away syringes, put away Methadone, or pick up a gun from my father . . . I mean, God knows what I would have done if I would have had to live through what my kids have lived through. So with that, I commend them.

What was it like for you?

For me? Being a wife?

Being a drug addict and getting better.

For me it was all new doors opening. I never had determination that I could be anything but a housewife. I always had insecurities that when I recovered, that when I went to a job, that nobody was going to accept me. I never even thought that I could do any job, let alone the one I'm doing now. It took me years to get that self-esteem back. And I wouldn't give it up for anybody. I've got it now. I've got the motivation that no matter what comes, how hard it may be. . . .

And that was as recently as four years ago?

Four years ago and then prior to that was on and off relapses where I would catch myself. Because I always saw myself as in control of the drug. I'll do it this week and next week I won't do it, then I'll do it the week after. So I always thought I was in control. My last relapse made me understand I wasn't in control. I walked around with the pills like it was my life, with the pills by me. I had to know that I had it there when I needed it. The hardest thing was that I needed it close to me. I could not go and get a job unless I took pills early in the morning. I could not put the kids on the school bus unless I took pills early in the morning. So every time I used to have to do something, either see a teacher or go to a job interview, I could not function without that. It became a part of me.

And the pills were Valium?

It was Valiums and alcohol. I started doing both because with the Valiums, it would take a longer time. But with the alcohol, it would zoom it up. It would be like a rush. But then besides that came the blackouts. The blackouts weren't that bad as long as there were people there so I could ask them, "What did I do? Did I sleep with anyone? Tell me." I couldn't remember bits and pieces that I did. That scared me too.

But I think the worst thing that scared me was that when I went back and told the doctor that it wasn't doing anything for me, that

I was still crying—rather than him sitting me down and asking me, "Well, let's go through your life and let's see why you feel so depressed, let's talk about it," what he did was he gave me twenty minutes of his time and said, "Okay, well that's not doing anything, let me up the milligrams." So I went back home and took the second dosage he gave me, which was not seventy-five no more, it was a hundred and fifty milligrams of Valium. To the point where my oldest daughter came home and asked me one day, "Where's Jachlyne?" "She went to sleep over her friend's house." "Whose house?" "I don't know." "You gave her permission not knowing the girl, not knowing where the girl lives. You just went along and gave her permission?" And then my daughter finally found the pills and said, "You know that quack that I've been taking you to every week? He's not helping you, he's drugging you and you're too stupid to see it." I said, "I can't cope. You don't understand, you don't understand how my life is going. *You don't understand. I'm on welfare,* I can't give you kids the proper way of life. Your father is running around with a twenty-one-year-old girl. He thinks nothing of you kids." And my daughter said, "Yeah? Keep taking them. You think you have no one now? You're going to see how you're going to be, all kind of lonesome. We've got one person in the family that's drugging, we don't need two." She took my pills and threw them across the yard, and I saw myself crawl after them and count them and put them back in the bottle. When I saw that, my kids, when I looked up and saw them looking at me, saying, "How pitiful you've gotten," I think that was the hair that broke the camel's back. I said that no matter how hard it is I'm going to get well.

I stayed home. I still have a hard time pulling up the shades. I lived in total darkness. I didn't want the sunlight in. With the pills, it brings you . . . I wouldn't say hallucinations, but it brings you very, very insecure, that you're afraid that someone might be looking in—that paranoia. My daughter still will get up on a Saturday and say, "Ma, you have to let the sunlight in." And I catch myself sometimes and say, "You know what? I want to see the sunlight because I've been in total darkness for so long."

How long did it take you to get off of them?

It took me mentally and physically three months. I went through the withdrawal in my house. I had my kids with me who would go

to school and they would each take turns coming home and baby-
sitting me, literally babysitting me. Because if they weren't there, I
was still going to try to keep that appointment with the doctor. To
this day, I still fight it. I know me. I know that my biggest weakness
is pills. That if I take 'em, I'll like 'em and I won't know when to
stop. For my back I've got a prescription for Motrin 600 that I haven't
filled for the simple reason that if I do fill it, and all I need is one,
I'm going to be on a roll. So what I do is, I fight it. I've got the
pain but I can stand it.

*Do you go to a Spanish-speaking meeting or do you go to regular A.A.
or . . . ?*

No, I don't go to A.A. or N.A. What I do is I go to church and
that to me is my A.A. and my N.A. I work the steps just like I work
my ten commandments. I try to follow the rules. As long as I keep
those twelve steps and the ten commandments, I feel that I can't go
wrong.

Maybe you could call me the oddball. I try to reach out to these
people and give them hope, give them some type of tomorrow, give
them spiritual hope. Since they're getting A.A. and N.A. from the
other counselors, what I try to do is get them to believe in something
higher than themselves.

Aren't they going to miss you?

I'll take them with me to Florida, the memories. I don't want to
do detox anymore. It's been rewarding, it's been excellent for me.
It has helped me in my sobriety, it has done wonders for my sobriety.
But it also puts a stress, seeing repeaters. At first it would be, "Okay,
where did I go wrong? Maybe there was something I missed that I
will do this time."

So I want to work with outpatients, I want to work with families.
Bring families together. Letting the spouses know that you love them
and I can't tell you if it's going to take one detox or maybe two or
maybe three, what I want to let you know is how the disease concept
works. And how you have to work your own group too and their
group is Al-Anon. Not to be codependent. Because I was codepen-

dent. I was a big, big enabler. To me it was, we'll go to one program and he'll get clean and we'll live happily ever after running off in the sunset. It really didn't turn out like that.

Did you leave him in New York?

No. I helped him here. He served some time in jail. I let him sleep here, not as husband and wife, but as someone caring for someone else. I tried to make him work his program, but he chose to go the other way. For me, to be healthy was to let go and pray that someday he'll find himself because I wasn't doing any benefit to him. What I was doing was every time he fell, I'd pick up the pieces. It was taking me down. It took the better part of me down. So what I do right now is, me and my kids talk about him constantly. He's in our prayers. That someday he'll be able to lick that problem, be able to find a way, and when he does, his family will be there for him. Me, as a wife, as an ex-wife, caring? Yes. As a future wife? No. As a good, good friend? Yes. We grew up together, we were childhood sweethearts. He taught me a lot that I have to be thankful for, the good and the bad. He gave me three beautiful kids that I have to be thankful for. We can't help it about his disease. One day hopefully he'll come around.

I had a sister that was hooked on Methadone for six years. I spoke to her counselors and her doctors and they felt that she wasn't ready to stop. I felt that she was ready. I felt that they weren't even looking at her as a human being. They were looking at her as, *every day that she comes into this clinic to pick up her methadone, it's two thousand dollars,* it keeps this clinic open. So to them, she would have never been ready. I took her to Long Island with me. At that time I had a ten room house. I did her detox. I went and bought Methadone on the street. I bought Valiums in the street and I was going to detox her. She tried to escape and go back to New York and then I did the worst detox. I tied her to a chair, I babysat her. We were linked together if she had to go to the bathroom. I spoon-fed her. It was thirty days. My sister's been clean since. My sister was, she's my baby sister, she was thirty at the time. She looked like she was fifty by the time the Methadone got through with her. She aged tremendously, because Methadone does age you eventually. It might not be now, but keep taking it and you'll see. And that's what it did to

her. She was skinny, she was withdrawn. Her cheeks, she had no
cheeks. Self-esteem, forget it. She didn't even care if she took a bath
a week ago. Once I cleaned her up, bought her normal clothes, my
sister started caring about herself again. Finally, we finally got my
sister back, the sister that we lost for so many years through heroin
and through Methadone. My sister saw her son die, and . . . "Well,
I'll be back to the funeral parlor but I've got to go cop first." The
death of her son . . . some people have a rock bottom? That wasn't
even her rock bottom, her eleven-year-old son dying. Being in a
funeral parlor, she had to go cop because she couldn't stand up. I
took her two kids away. That wasn't even her rock bottom. Facing
me in court and me taking her two children away, *that* wasn't even
her rock bottom. After a while I started thinking she had no rock
bottom. What's it going to take to make this girl change?

Do you think that some people have no bottom?

No. I have to believe everybody has a bottom. I've seen people
sleeping in the streets. I did it too, and that wasn't even my rock
bottom. It was all right sleeping on the benches in New York, sleeping in hallways in New York—that wasn't my rock bottom. My
rock bottom was when my kids looked at me and said, "You call
yourself a mother? Please, you're a pitiful one." And then me looking
at them and saying, "If I'm doing it and he's doing it, God, where
are they going to be? It's not their fault."

Do you worry about them getting into drugs?

No, I think that worry's over. My twenty-year-old proved it. She
was on a mission for two years on cocaine.

After you got clean?

After I got clean. I cried. That didn't do anything. I talked to her.
That didn't do anything. Talked about her dad. That didn't do anything. Her dad came over and talked to her and *that* didn't do anything. It was when she saw the boy that she loves, who is the baby's

father, when she saw him take the food money and leave her baby
without food, without Pampers, just to get his cocaine, *that* woke
her up. She said, "If he's doing that, I might someday do that and
leave my daughter without food just to get my high. To feed my
high, it's not worth it." She says she carries that with her every day.
She says "I think Dad taught me a good lesson because every time
I got high, I kept saying, you could be like your daddy if you don't
get a hold of yourself now." Now she can be in a place and see
people doing lines and all she does is get her coat and leave. She
doesn't want to be around it. She says she still feels herself getting
nervous. "I don't know what the nerves are from. Maybe it's from
fear that if they keep offering it, that I might just say, yeah, why
not? 'Cause I know when they bring out the coke that the sweat,
the shivers are there and I have to put my coat on and run." I've got
a son-in-law who I sent to N.A. I gave up Valiums, I gave up the
alcohol, and this (cigarette) I know eventually I'll give up. It's just
going to be a slow process like the rest of it. I used to be going to
parties saying I gave up alcohol, but once somebody offered it to
me I would drink it. Now I can finally say, "I'll stay thirsty." I
won't drink it. That's something.

The Hispanic community seems very closed. . . .

A lot of them have a lot of pride. The Hispanic people, they're
raised that if you do that, you're a bad woman, you're a bad mother.
Sometimes you get disowned from the family completely.

By admitting it?

Mmhmm. So a lot of them keep it in the closet. I have a lot of
patients come in and say, "My mother must never find out I was in
a place like this." To me, I think it would be better to tell, but to
them, no.

Why did you agree to let me talk to you?

Me, I have nothing to hide. I give myself a commendation because
I went through all this and can sit here and tell the story and have

people see the success of it all. And every day to me it's like I've come so far that now I want it to be known. I tell my story and a lot of people can't picture it. I tell it to people and people say, "No, not you." I say, "Yes, the woman that you see here has done everything that you can think of. That doesn't make me a bad person. I don't regret it. It's my life. I don't want to do it again. I don't ever want to do it again, but I'm not ashamed of it. I think in a way maybe it was a benefit to me, it made me the person I am today with the values that I have. Without what I went through, maybe I would have been a close-minded person."

I've had a lot of people say, "I've had the sobriety, but I was still miserable." I think that along with the sobriety, you also have to be able to find yourself. It is a long, dragged-out process. You look, and you see that it may never come, and after a while you start giving up hope. And you go back because you say, "God, I've had a year, nothing has changed, I'm still living in poverty, I'm still eating shit, I'm still answering to welfare, I haven't gotten a job, and you told me that sobriety would be *beautiful*."

It is, but you've got to feel it within, not on the outside. It's got to be all over you.

November 1990

Part Two

Abuse

I hate words like darling, baby, sweetheart,
and phrases like God bless you—and people
who beg for love, or who propose bed or who
with sweet kisses and weak looks try to
advance their interests—it's like a disease
oozing its smeary infection. I can only be had
by my own consent, by wordless violence
that is natural to me...no matter how
hurtful—or how brutal.

—Ludwig Bemelmans,
writing as the
unnamed woman in
*Are You Hungry Are
You Cold*

Katie

An only child, Katie is twenty-seven years old. She has been married and divorced twice. She lives with two of her young children; her first husband has custody of their oldest boy. She has an apartment in a small college town in New England where her father runs a convenience store. While in junior high school she was described as "cute"; now she is striking. Although thin, she claims, "but I need to lose weight. Food is another addiction." She puts herself down, catches herself, rolls her eyes and shakes her head. She continues to grieve the death of her mother. Katie began drinking at eleven, and controlling her drinking while still in high school. She stays at home with her children and lives on welfare. She has been continuously sober since 1988.

The first time I drank I was eleven. I spent a lot of time alone. My mother came home early one night and she had some little bottles of champagne. I had never asked her before if I could have anything to drink. I just assumed the answer would be no. I asked her that night and she said that it was all right. She put a little bit in a glass for me and I drank it. I loved it. I just felt all warm and comforted. I was in the kitchen and I remember she walked in, took one look at me and said, "I think you've had enough."

She took the champagne away from me and she put it in the refrigerator. I remember thinking, "No, I want it. Don't take it away." I spent a lot of time by myself at home and the house was full of booze and there was nobody there.

When I was twelve years old I drank at home, alone, just about every day. I have a friend whose father died years ago of alcoholism, so she knew about it. She would call and say, "So, what are you doing?" and I'd say, "Well, I'm sitting in the pantry again." That's where we kept the booze. I would sit in the pantry and drink. She'd tell me I was an alcoholic. I'd say, "I am not an alcoholic. I'm only twelve, I can't be an alcoholic."

How much were you drinking then?

Whatever it took. I remember watering down the booze, the stuff that my parents didn't drink. When I was twenty my parents were camping. I went up to their camp one night and I cracked a half-gallon of Seagram's. I was the only one drinking out of that bottle. I went up to a different campsite where I drank some vodka. The next morning when I got up, my mother brought me over to the bottle and said, "You were the only one drinking out of this bottle." There was only about an inch left in it. So I had a huge tolerance. I would stop drinking altogether for a while, and with just one wine cooler I could feel a buzz. Then, before I knew it, I was right back into drinking like a pig.

Towards the end I couldn't feel oblivion again. I was in a lot of pain. I was willing to do anything, anything at all, to escape what I was feeling.

Which was what? What was the pain?

Oh, God. Rage. Just rage. A couple of weeks before my son was born my husband told me that he had a girlfriend. I hadn't been drinking throughout the pregnancy but I picked up; that was it. I was pregnant with my youngest son. I really thought I could have a drink with dinner. That didn't work. I ended up getting hammered. My son was a month old when I got sober and it was two weeks before he was born that I picked up. That was hell.

Did you have all three kids with the same man?

No, the two younger ones.

I got pregnant when I was in high school during one of my not drinking times. I was with this guy, he was my addiction. It was awful. He was real abusive but it wasn't as important for me not to get *beat up* as it was to hold onto him. In a two-year period, from when I was sixteen to when I was almost eighteen, I had tried to commit suicide, I had run away to Georgia, and I had gotten pregnant.

It's so stupid, when you're kids, you know. He was seventeen, I was sixteen. We had four hundred dollars and we thought, "Hey, we're rich. We can go live with this money." We took off in his car. We thought that it was my parents' fault, his parents' fault, everybody else's fault why our relationship was the way it was. So we took off with this big four hundred dollars and headed down south. We figured we'd go to Florida where it was warm. We got to Georgia and we had forty bucks, an empty gas tank, empty stomachs. We were in the most disgusting motel room I've ever seen in my life. You could hear the cockroaches. It was really gross. This guy that I thought was supposed to be taking care of me just sat there on the bed and cried. He wanted to go home, he'd had enough. I just figured he was a wimp. I was still gonna stay. I was still willing to go for it. But I ended up calling my father up and he said, "You better get your ass up here. There's going to be an APB out on you. . . . " I didn't want to go home. But we did and I was put on probation.

Did you marry him?

Yes. I've been married twice. I don't even remember if that was before or after I tried to kill myself. It was within months anyway. He beat me up again and again and I just hated myself. I didn't think that there was anything good about me. I didn't think that I deserved for anybody to care about me so I couldn't believe that anybody did.

I was supposed to be going to school. Instead I went down to my father's store, had breakfast there and went back home again. My grandparents had died years before, but their medicines were still there. There were three medicine cabinets full of drugs. And that day I ate them all. I thought if I was going to die, at least I'd be buzzed out before I went. Just go to sleep and not wake up. That's really what I wanted. My father came home at lunch time, he came home early and I was really out of it. He took me to the hospital.

They wanted me to drink Ipecac and I said, "No," and they said, "You're either going to drink this or get your stomach pumped and believe me, you'd rather drink this." There was this really mean nurse in there and I said, "Okay." I drank it and I was in ICU for a while.

I was embarrassed that it didn't work. People heard about it. These girls in school came up to me one day just laughing and said, "Why don't you go and commit suicide?" "I would if I thought I could do it right." That was my attitude. It was awful. I just stayed with the guy, and I ended up getting pregnant. Nobody thought I'd graduate from high school because I was pregnant. I didn't care about having a diploma then. But they said I couldn't do it, so I *had* to do it. We got married during winter vacation.

What made you decide to stop drinking?

Well, actually I didn't even know I had 'til I had been sober for awhile. The second marriage broke up. I got drunk. I was drinking and drinking and drinking and the pain wouldn't go away. I had all this anger and I just stuffed it. I just wouldn't let it show. I'd be smiling, and an outside person would say, "You are handling this really, really well." I would just smile and say, "Yes, I am. Thank you." And then I'd go and get drunk. I accepted all of the responsibility for the problems in that marriage. It was so apparent to me that it was all my fault. I hated myself and I went in and out of really obsessing, thinking I loved my husband and hating his girlfriend, really hating her, just literally hating her, wanting her dead.

I was coming back from the bar one day and my husband and his girlfriend and her daughter and my kids were all walking down the street like a happy family. I just snapped, that was it. I was in my car, I was drunk and I put my foot down on the accelerator and I came about five feet away. . . . All I saw was her at that point. It was the whole family, but I only saw her. I believed if I just wiped her out then I could go back, to my place in the family, and everything would be fine. At the last minute I remember thinking, "I don't want to go to jail, and I don't want to go to hell either." I turned the wheel, kept going down the street. The trees were looking real inviting. I wanted to ram into one of those trees and just end it. I didn't have any self-worth at all. I had no self-respect. My whole self was Steven's wife, the kids' mother. There was nothing else to me. I was everyone else's me. The suicide went through my head. "Okay, this person will get over it, that person will get over it." My daughter, Amy, was only two. I figured she'd forget me. My youngest one didn't know me. He was only a month old and I wasn't really even there for him during that month. I was drinking. Then I came across my oldest son who had had some real severe emotional problems. He'd been abused in every way that a human being can be abused. I knew that he couldn't get over my death. If I killed myself I knew that I'd be killing a part of him too.

I headed back to the bar. That idea was blown. I had to escape from all this shit. I drank and drank. It wouldn't work, it just didn't work anymore. In the beginning when I drank, if I was depressed, I'd come up. If I was tense, I'd get calm. It would always get me sort of feeling middle-ground, or not feeling at all. And it just didn't work anymore. Still, still, I couldn't figure out that I was an alcoholic. I was still in denial after all that. But one thing was clear to me: I had some real mental health problems. "I'm nuts, I'm crazy." I knew, I could see, finally, that this was really irrational. Being homicidal and suicidal is not a rational thing.

I had an appointment with my son's school psychologist the next day and I went to her office and I just told her the truth. I told her what was going on. I said, "I really need help." So she sent me to a psychiatrist. I talked to him and asked him if there was a place I could go to rest. I told him, "I don't want to go to Northampton State Hospital or any place like that. I just want to go someplace where I can rest." So he set me up at Noble Hospital psych ward.

I went there and the first thing I walked into there was a self-esteem group. There were these pieces of paper and we had to write down three things that we liked about ourselves and I sat there and I cried because the only thing I could come up with was that I loved God. I couldn't think of anything good about me. They said for me not to worry about it. I stayed there for a while, and I told them the truth. I told them what I was doing. I told them about the stuff with Steven and Jill. I told them that all I could think of to do was to get as drunk as I could as fast as I could.

They sent me to an A.A. meeting. A counselor asked me, "Do you think you're an alcoholic?" And I said, "Well, you know, maybe I'm a borderline alcoholic. I could be if I let myself be." A lot of denial. He said, "Why don't you check out an A.A. meeting?" It's like, "No, I don't think so." I envisioned a bunch of old guys in trench coats sitting around drinking coffee talking about how bad life was without booze. I was very wrong about that. He said I needed to go to one meeting. After that it was my choice, but I had to go to one meeting. There were a few other people in the ward who were also to attend the meeting.

We cracked all these stupid jokes on the way down. I was so scared. I would use laughter as another mask. Cracking these stupid jokes like, "Why don't we just blow this off and go to the package store." I got there and I was still making these dumb jokes. But this one was serious, *"This would be a lot easier to do if I had a shot in me."*

I went in and I was listening to the speaker. He was talking about sleeping on the railroad tracks and all this stuff that didn't apply to me. I listened and thought, "This isn't so bad. Thank God, I'm not an alcoholic." The last thing he said was, "If you think you've got your drinking under control, then at some time or another it must have been out of control." And that hit me. It reminded me of a period of my life that I call the grey life, because I don't know what happened, it's so blurry. It was a period of four years that I have very little memory of. I remembered how hard I drank then. I was really into drugs also. I'd been controlling it after that, or so I thought. I knew that at some point or another I must've been *out* of control. The speaker was funny, and there were some nice looking guys there, and I thought, "Well, this is it. I'll go to these meetings and find a nice sober guy and everything will be wonderful. Oh boy."

Did you go to A.A. and just stop?

Yeah. I haven't had a drink since before I went into the hospital. It was two years ago, June 7, 1988. That's incredible. I can't imagine me not drinking for that long.

A.A. worked?

Well, sort of. I was going to the meetings, but my priority was definitely the kids. Any time I had left over was for A.A., which was not very much time when you have little ones. So I would bring the kids to meetings with me. That wasn't working out too good. I was going to meetings and listening but I didn't have a clue as to what the hell was going on. I thought, "What are these people talking about?" Somehow I managed in my head to make all my problems A.A.'s fault. "If it wasn't for this stupid A.A. business I would be with my husband now."

It was really frustrating with the kids. I knew I needed to be at meetings. I knew there were a lot of things I needed to be doing. In A.A. they said follow suggestions and I couldn't do that. They said to go to thirty meetings in thirty days, sixty in sixty, ninety in ninety and I couldn't get a babysitter. I might've gotten a babysitter twice a week. I would bring the kids to meetings and I would be focusing more on keeping them quiet so everyone else could listen than listening myself.

It just wasn't working. I was sober about six months and then I wanted to drink again. I really wanted to drink. Before a meeting, I wanted to drink. During a meeting, I wanted to drink. After a meeting, I wanted to drink. It took me five months before I got a sponsor. I asked a lot of people. "I'll be your friend, I can't be your sponsor . . ." There's not a lot of women who are sober long enough to be a good sponsor. Certainly not around here. There's not a lot of women that are sober and the ones that are have X amount of sponsees already and they can only give so much.

One night I was at a business meeting. I had a home group and this group was the most accepting of my children. During the business meeting they were arguing about what to do about kids in general. But I knew it was my kids. I was thinking, "Fuck this. Forget it. I can't do this. I'm just going to shut myself in my house and isolate, go out to buy bread and milk." Then it was like, "I can't do that. I can't do this. I can't do any of this. I can't live. I can't drink. I can't not drink. I can't be a mom." I just couldn't stand it. I couldn't stand me and I couldn't stand my life. That was it. I made up my mind. I was going to kill myself. Again. Sober. The same stuff.

Five people followed me home from that business meeting. Five people came to my house to make sure I was okay. To talk to me. I thought, "This is real." It was amazing that people really did care about me. And it wasn't the people who I had expected to care about me. It was these strangers, these alcoholic people, who are just trying to not drink. They cared about me and they knew that I was in trouble. I didn't even say anything, but they came. It really touched me. I started to want to stay alive again.

The next day the chairman of the group, who was one of the five people, stopped by my house. He said that he and his wife would take care of my kids for a couple of weeks so I could go to treatment. There was an EAP [employee assistance program] guy where he worked and he got me set up into treatment.

I went to the Brattleboro Retreat. My recovery didn't start until I got there. That was the best thing I ever did for myself. I was real fortunate to have insurance. A lot of people don't have insurance and that bothers me. . . .

When you step away from something and look at it, you can see it better. That's what happened with my life when I was in treatment, I stepped out of it and then I could see it. And it was a mess. It was a real mess. No wonder I wanted to kill myself. I could see what I was doing to my kids. I thought I was staying there for my kids and doing all this stuff for my kids. I had to choose. I had to choose to go back to doing the same things and probably end up dying, or to take care of myself. I voluntarily placed my kids in foster care. I stayed in treatment for the six weeks.

I came home and I went to a halfway house for a few months. I graduated from there. Then I had to go to a shelter because where I lived before was not a healthy place for me to be. It's just down the street from my father. He was my landlord. He worked downstairs and he lived next door. He was real codependent and it just wasn't healthy. Not to mention the fact that it was too small. DSS wouldn't let me have my kids back with an apartment that small. It was cockroach infested. I mean, I had threatened my own father with the Board of Health. I couldn't live like that. It was really not a good place for me to be. It was haunted with memories. So from the halfway house I went to a shelter and I got a nice apartment and I got my kids back.

A year ago my oldest son started a fire. One of the things he was doing was setting fires and he had to be hospitalized. It was just really screwy. There was a 51A* put on me, from DSS, for abusing my children, which didn't happen. Sad story. I got that all cleared up. For awhile I couldn't see my kids. I wasn't sure I was ever going to see them again, for something that I didn't even do. They left my

*A report from the Department of Social Services for neglect and abuse.

house. There were no marks on them whatsoever, there was nothing wrong with them. The next day, when they brought them to the doctor's, there were no marks on them. But somehow, in between point A and point B, there was a 51A put on myself and my boyfriend for abuse. But there were witnesses. . . . It was crazy. It was like a bomb went off in my house or something. It was just . . . aaahhh. I couldn't handle it.

There was an investigation. They couldn't prove anything so I got my kids back last February. In January, my mother was diagnosed as having cancer. She died in August. It was a hard time. There's been a lot of good stuff and that's what keeps me going through the bad times. Before, there were really no good times. There was excitement and danger and all that stuff but not like . . . I remember when my kids came back. When they told me my kids were coming back I was talking to my sponsor on the phone and I was crying and I asked her, "Why am I crying? My kids are coming back." She had to tell me what this is, that this feeling is called joy. And with this feeling, joy, you cry sometimes. But it's not sad tears, it's happy tears, it's joy. Wow. I didn't know that feeling.

I understand myself a lot more now. I understand a lot of my crazy behavior that I just couldn't before. I've had flashbacks of things that happened to me when I was a little girl. That was the purpose of alcohol, to forget all that.

It took about two years for that stuff to start coming up but it did. It was painful at the time, but it was worth feeling that way to see why my behavior was, and sometimes is, the way it is. It helps me to accept myself more. To know that it's not because I'm stupid. It's because I was hurt.

What kinds of things?

I was sexually abused by three of my relatives when I was little, real little. My mother abused me verbally and . . . spiritually. I don't know if technically there is such a thing, but there must be, because I lived in it. See, this is hard. It's hard for me right now to say things that my mother did to me because I'm grieving. It doesn't mean I love her any less, but there was a time in her life, right after her parents died, and I don't know why or how, but she was spiritually very sick and she abused me. So my perspective became twisted.

She was very angry. You know anger is a normal part of grieving and she didn't have any of the help that I have. And that's when she was violent towards me.

It was mostly emotional. I had everything material. Anything that I wanted. I didn't have things like encouragement. Or even another being. I started working when I was nine. After school I would go to work and then I would go home and be alone. I went to bed and they would come home late, so there was nobody home. I felt like I was in a cage, and the way I escaped from that was with alcohol.

A lot of people know me pretty well. My sponsor knows all about me. All of it. A lot of it's still a mystery, but it comes to me in little bits. What I can handle at the time is what I get. Sometimes it doesn't feel that way. This grieving stuff is . . . ooohhh. It's awful sometimes, it's really awful. Sometimes my feelings feel too big for me. But it usually only lasts a day. I don't think I can handle it but I hang in and the next day's a little bit better.

The holidays are coming up. I have a hard time with holidays. I want my mother. I do not want to have dinner Thanksgiving day with my father and however many of my kids can be there. But I'm making things change. I invited some friends to come for dinner, too. That way my father won't give me any grief. If they're his buddies or whatever, I'm a moving target. But if a friend of mine is there, he won't do it.

Relationships are still hard. I don't like nice guys very much. I get bored real quick. This guy I'm sort of seeing, we've been in and out of a relationship for a year. He's real nice, you know. He's helpful and thoughtful and all this stuff and I get freaked out. I get just so close and then I think, I'm not going through round three. I guess I don't want to get hurt again. I back off. Then it's like, "What are you doing, Katie? Don't be stupid." And I go back again. He's a nice guy. Once he referred to me as a bitch. Once, in a year. I let him know that that was *not* okay to do, don't do it again. It crossed my boundaries and all these things and words that I didn't know existed. I didn't know there were such things as boundaries. But I know it now. Now I can say "You're crossing a boundary. Please don't do that again. I don't like it."

What would you say to a woman who is still drinking?

If you can't stop drinking, go to meetings until you can learn how to stop drinking or want to stop drinking. You don't have to be sober to go to A.A. You go to A.A. to learn how to be sober. I didn't really want to stop drinking either. What alcoholic really wants to stop drinking, for God's sake? It's more like a "have to." You get to a point where you *have to*.

Sobriety kind of grows on you?

   It does. At A.A. they say, "If you don't get A.A., it'll get you." It's true. 'Cause I went for a long time and I didn't get it. I just couldn't grasp any of it. And then, I got some. It seems funny because sometimes it seems like I still don't get it. I know that I'm not drinking, and I know that I'm alive, and those are two big things. Something I tell myself, especially when I see friends and family who are still drinking, "If you're breathing, there's hope."
   Wouldn't it be nice if society as a whole could see that? Then you wouldn't be judged for having a disease. If I had cancer, they'd be, "Oh, poor Katie has cancer, what can I do for you?" But I have alcoholism and so people back off.
   If I try to look for the goodness in people, and even active drunks have goodness in them, then I'd say living isn't so bad.

November 1990

Mary

A tall and physically fit fifty-year-old, she stopped drinking in 1976; ten years later she gave up all drugs. "I grew up in an alcoholic home in Westchester County, New York. Very upper class." Because her life improved so much after she got sober, she belittles herself for having wasted so much time. She attends both Narcotics Anonymous and Alcoholics Anonymous. A cab driver in Key West, she goes to college at night. Her son Sean, now grown, is about to go into the navy, leaving her alone for the first time in eighteen years. I interviewed her by telephone.

At thirteen I really started drinking. I had a fantasy of escaping. I wanted to live like children in Africa in huts, or children in England on barges. I fantasized about being in those places, never where I was. I always fantasized; I still do. I look at clouds and think they're mountains. On the playground I would always be off behind a tree somewhere. I was happy to be left alone. We moved a lot so it was real easy to be that way. If you weren't in a clique or the teacher didn't pick on you, it was easy to disappear.

My father would be unable to get out of bed because of cirrhosis of the liver. In and out of the hospital. Hitting my mother, trying to hit me. My mother would go in the bedroom and cry. Cry and cry and cry. I decided to protect my mother against my father. I think I was really angry at her for never defending herself. Finally she got up the courage to divorce him. I was drinking.

I remember the weekend when I became aware that alcohol was

my answer. I was in school and I had a D average in biology. In New York they have Regents exams. At the end of each year you can read one review book and you can go in and take the Regents exam and pass the course for the year. I took some beer up to my room and started drinking beer and studying. I stayed up all night, drinking beer and smoking cigarettes. I was about thirteen and I got one of the highest grades in the course. I decided that alcohol made me smarter. It wasn't the fact that I studied. I decided alcohol made me smarter and it was my little secret.

One day I got really drunk. I drank a whole fifth of gin and took my friends out in a jeep. I got into an accident. Going down a hill, I went head on into our barn, through the windshield, and ended up in the hospital. Another boy did also. It was a pretty bad accident. I was in the hospital and my mother thought it had happened with this boyfriend of mine who had a motorcycle. I said to her, "But I was drunk." Over and over and no one listened to me. They laughed. They must have been able to smell it on me. I had a little fracture in my skull. They kept giving me lollipops. I was so young.

My mother decided that I ought to live with my aunt and uncle out in California, so I moved out to Laguna Beach. That was the beginning of a real free-for-all because they're quite wealthy. They were always gone. I had a cousin my age and she and I just lived there with housekeepers. We would get drunk and stoned in Tijuana. I was fifteen, going to school drunk every day. The friends I met were surfers and kids that had dropped out of school. Nobody really took control.

I came back to Westchester and lived with my mother for my senior year in high school. I have no idea how I made it through high school. I was so drunk at graduation they almost didn't let me go up to get my diploma. I immediately moved, after graduation, to New York City, to Greenwich Village. I knew New York pretty well. I worked at Lord & Taylor's. My father is from around Riverside Drive. He went to Columbia. I loved the city. I still do.

I drank a lot. I didn't do anything great. I moved into an apartment in the Village. I had many jobs. I usually couldn't keep a job for very long, or didn't want to. I worked in coffee houses. I parked cars on 42nd Street. I'd take the subway all the way down. I think about that now. At 2 A.M. I'd be on the subway. I'd see things: people getting in fights, and sometimes people would come up to me and I'd get out of it. I was just really lucky, I guess. I never felt adequate.

I would meet nice guys, but I wouldn't be interested in them. I moved in with a guy who was a junkie, a heroin addict. He was a cab driver. He was really bright and he was a writer. Everybody was a writer or an actor. You know, the beatnik era. I loved going to the clubs. I did everything for him. I just—did everything for him. I cleaned and cooked, I copped for him. Occasionally I would meet somebody nice. I would always reject him. I was really obsessive over that guy.

Sometimes I would just get up and travel across the country. I hitchhiked to California. I went and put my thumb out and rode trucks out to L.A. and looked up my cousin. I was too wild to be anywhere around my uncle and aunt at that time.

I lived in a really sleazy hotel and worked on the strip. I'd do anything. I worked in bars. I got drunk. I was doing drugs, mostly doing a lot of speed. Mostly speed and alcohol. Not any heroin, not . . . much. I never got into heroin that much. There was something in me that didn't want to use needles. It was the culture surrounding it that I didn't like although I liked guys that were on it.

At one point when I was drinking a lot I worked at a bar in North Hollywood. The bar was owned by Jerry Colonna's brother, the comedian. All the girls in there were hooking and I wasn't. I was supporting my boyfriend and I wasn't doing that yet. The manager of the bar said there were two guys coming in who had paid for me. I was going to have to be with them. He had already arranged it. They were lawyers and I was supposed to sleep with both of them. I was like, "Wait a minute," but I met them. We went out and I started drinking martinis as fast as I could. I got up, said I was going to the ladies' room and slipped out the back door.

Well, I don't know if what happened next was related or not, but the next night I was on my way home from work, and a guy jumped out of the bushes and beat the shit out of me. I fought him and I was a mess. I was black and blue. I went home, walked upstairs, went into the bathroom and slit my wrists. I was thinking, "This room, this place . . . " I hit an artery and ran outside in the hallway; the blood was spurting. Someone called an ambulance and took me to the hospital. An orderly told me I'd committed suicide wrong. I was supposed to slit my wrist *down* my vein.

The minute I got out of that hospital I went and bought a bottle of vodka and put it in my duffle bag. I flew home. Left the boyfriend, left everything. The owner of the hotel took me for a drive before he took me to the airport. He drove me all through Beverly Hills and other affluent places and said, "This is where you should be. You shouldn't be living where you're living." The funny thing is . . . that was my background. My uncle owned a big office building in L.A. And I thought, "This is where I should be? This doesn't impress me either." And I flew back. I moved back into the city and just drank. I smoked a lot of pot and did pills: Valium, sleeping pills, speed. I just spent a lot of years knocking around. I would go back and forth to L.A.

I started going down to Florida, which was where my father was living. I went down to see him, went to the beach and decided it was a great lifestyle—everybody drinking and partying. LSD and acid started coming out. I was a good swimmer: instant job. I taught swimming on the beach in community pools and partied all the time and by that time my father was like the town drunk. He would be in the streets drunk, beaten up, and he'd come up and yell at me in front of people.

I had started sailing. I met some people who were starting a development down in the Turks and Caicos islands and did I want to go? I said sure. We bought an old freighter. I stayed there a year. The booze, it was Heineken, Mt. Gay rum. I didn't do drugs. They weren't around and most of these men were pretty well off. They called themselves the Seven Dwarves. I had one boyfriend. I did a lot of work on the boat, and just hung out. Now it's like a fancy jet set resort. But when we got there it was nothing. There was just this little settlement and the people there were so ignorant. If I said I was from Florida they said, "Oh, we know that island." They were so beautiful, but they were really exploited. They got paid twenty-five cents an hour to dig in coral rock. To build the hotel, the Third Turtle Inn.

I started sailing, mostly on crew boats bringing cargo back to the island. I went down to the Exumas and to St. Thomas. I would just bum around. Everybody had a plane. You could just go to an airstrip, they would land on the Selina Bins, and on the salt ponds, these hard sand flats. Everybody was drinking even when they were flying. Nobody cared, once you got out of the states, about regulations.

One time I was flying down to Mexico with a guy, they called him Pirate Jim. He gave a false flight plan. He told the FAA we were going to Georgia and we were really going to Mexico to buy some pot. I don't know what else he was buying. We're flying over the Gulf of Mexico at about eleven thousand feet and he passed out. He just started falling asleep. I said, "Jim." I woke him up and he said, "What's wrong?" And I'm like, "Please, I just want you to stay awake while you're flying a plane." And he said, "It's on automatic pilot, it's no problem. Take a nap, you know."

We flew to Cozumel, then rented another plane. We flew way into the Yucatan. There were these fields with marijuana growing so tall, taller than I am, tall. We landed in the fields, met a guy who had something to do with the government, I don't know what he was. We'd make a connection, fly right back into Ft. Lauderdale or Naples and unload. I mean the plane must have smelled. This was like before people were really hot after drugs. It was so easy and such quick money. I was twenty-six.

Then I started coming down to Key West. I'd been down to Key West a couple of times. I was drinking and I met a lot of people sailing. They were smugglers, smuggling drugs and stuff and I was really attracted to them. This one guy I really liked used to bring in boatloads of pot. He always had a lot of money and we started going down to Key West a lot. So I got to know people there.

I decided I was going to start surfing. I'd go to Juno Beach and surf. I always wanted to go surfing in Hawaii and one day we had all this money, $25,000 in cash, and just took off and went to Hawaii. I had a Mexican dress with the embroidery. I bought a pair of flip flops. I never was able to afford real shoes. I was never able to afford anything, even though there was all this money around. I couldn't even keep myself in rubber flip flops. I was always going barefoot. I walk around Key West today thinking, "How was I able to walk around barefoot?"

There was this other guy I flew with named Mike. We flew to Hawaii, via all these other cities. We flew to Houston and up to San Francisco and we flew to L.A. I remember waking up in hotel rooms wondering which city I was in.

We flew into Honolulu. Then we flew into Maui and by the time we got there, blew our money and ended up with $200 so we were just going to move up into the mountains and live. I got to know the island pretty well. I don't know where I got my energy. From drugs I guess. I'd run on the beach. I don't know what I thought. I had my world. I worked at night waitressing. I'd get fired and get another job.

So, at this point you had no idea drugs were dangerous. Or that what you were doing was—dubious?

I knew that what I was doing to get the drugs was wrong. When I needed drugs I would go downtown and I would do anything to get whatever drugs I needed. You know, I would go to bed with anybody. I would sell, (whispers), I don't want my son to hear this. I would sell myself. I had nothing, no personal possessions to sell. *God, my son.* I would sell myself.

I was meeting people. People that seemed to like me, and tried to give me breaks, but I would resort to prostitution. I remember one time I was sitting at this party at this guy's house. He was talking about me to everybody else as if I wasn't there. He was saying how he'd seen me begging on the streets and how I'd do anything for drugs. I'd give blow jobs and do anything . . . so that's the way people envisioned me.

I ended up meeting my son's father. We sailed a boat back from Hawaii together and I moved over to the mainland. It took us two months to sail the boat across the ocean, all the way to California, in the winter. We had to sail real far north to catch westerly winds. We sailed it into Santa Barbara and I was drinking even then. I was pregnant.

I went back east to Florida. I was doing a lot of drugs, mostly speed. This is when I got really bad. Speed, mescaline, and downs and drinking. I was pregnant. Then he got put in jail for a long time. There I was, in the streets. I was pretty much living on people's boats, pregnant. People took care of me all the time. A lot of people enabled me over the years. Older men would bail me out—keep me. People who had sailboats would let me watch their boats when they went away. The boat yards really took care of me the whole time I was pregnant, but I still drank. I had no concern for the baby. And yet I did. My son's father got out of jail and I moved up to northern Florida. He had bought a bar and said, "Why don't you go up there?" It was a real redneck part of Florida. In the boonies. And there I was about to deliver. I had my baby up there in Vero Beach. That's when

I really slid down and all of a sudden the paranoia, the fears, they were just awful . . . the depression. It's amazing that my son lived.

Sean was born six pounds, four ounces, and has always been in advanced classes, but he was born with belabored breathing and tremors. I was tripping the night I went into labor. That's when the drinking really got bizarre. . . . I got worse. I got worse, worse, worse, and moved back to Ft. Lauderdale.

I was a really neglectful mother. One night I took so many Tuinols, sleeping pills. I was on this person's boat. Sean was just a toddler. There was this little skinny gangplank, going up to the boat. If he had fallen in I could not have gotten him. I couldn't move, I had no coordination. I was watching him, thinking, "Please make it up that gangplank." I remember the feeling, that horrible feeling I had inside, that if he died it would be totally my fault. Totally my fault if he drowned. I just watched him. I tried to get up. I just had to be real silent and watch him. I was so scared, but he made it.

I started to get real paranoid and I started to have feelings of child abuse. I was terrified of Sean's father and friends. They were all smugglers. Smuggling wasn't like love and peace and pot. People I knew were being killed, people were getting ripped off. Everybody carried a gun around. People started stashing stuff in my apartment. His friends came down, giving me all these drugs to sell. To help me? I was getting deeper and deeper into drugs, more paranoid, and totally neglectful. It's just a miracle, just a miracle that the boy's life was saved.

Somehow I got an apartment. I guess I was on welfare. We had no furniture. I don't know what I ever fed him—my son. Mostly he was still breastfeeding, weaning himself. I loved him, too. I spent a lot of time with him. We do have a really good relationship. Everybody in the high school says, "You've got a great boy, how did you do it?" And I'm like, *If you only knew*.

I began having a fantasy of me being sober. It was me in these very proper clothes, because I used to wear these long skirts, whatever—rags. Me out wearing proper clothes, out selling boats, a yacht broker making lots of money and raising my son in this nice little town. I visualized a town on Cape Cod. I remember thinking it was impossible.

By this time I was having nightmares from the drugs and the booze. I feared being a parent, having been brought up with such an abusive father. I was afraid I was going to abuse my son. I locked his bedroom door and then just sat up. . . . I used to sit up at night with a knife in my hand. I would hallucinate about people coming in the windows, or rats. The places I did live in did have rats, and Sean's father and everything around me were real reasons to be paranoid. I was afraid of standing up to them because I thought they might kill me.

That's the way my world was. I feared harming someone else. I would be looking at people and talking to them. On the outside I'd be real nice but on the inside I'd be wanting to tear them apart and kill them and I knew this was not normal. I went to a psychiatrist and he said I should go to A.A. I was really insulted.

One day I said, "I'm not going to drink today." I woke up in the morning and said, "I'll have just one glass of wine." I got so drunk. I drank the whole half gallon of wine. I passed out, woke up, and it was still only noon. My son was toddling around somewhere. I would go out, on a bicycle or something, and leave him alone in the apartment. I wouldn't remember leaving him alone. I would be in a black-out. I'd come back, and it would be dark and he'd be in there screaming.

I was always running. Running from Sean's father. Thinking I had to run from the police because they were going to take my son away.

One day I called A.A. I don't know why it came to my mind, but I called. They told me where the meeting was and I went to see this very wealthy man named Scott. I used to work on his boat. He took me to the meeting but I wasn't ready to hear anything. The mayor of Ft. Lauderdale was at the meeting. He and I had gotten drunk together. I felt so inferior to everybody else. Everyone looked so clean and so together. I still felt like I was crazier than everybody. I was more insane. I couldn't talk about it. So I went out and drank.

Scott decided that he was going to marry me. He gave me an engagement ring. I wasn't in love with him but everyone said, "Marry him, he's a millionaire." So I took his engagement ring and moved on his boat.

One day I got into an automobile accident. A real bad one. It was on Christmas Eve. They put me in jail and I had all these back tickets. They had a bench warrant for conspiracy for smuggling drugs because some people had given state's evidence against me. Scott came to bail me out and it was like $10,000 bail. There were two separate charges. One was a federal offense and one was for traffic tickets. I had no license and had all these tickets. Scott bailed me out. But I spent those three days in jail. It was Christmas.

I had been in jail before for public intoxication. One time I was in for five days. I had no way of being bailed out. Over the years I'd spent time in there and they used to put you in the drunk tank. It was a padded cell with a hole. That's where you threw up. That's where you shit and peed. There were others in there too. They had a little window where they would look in on you. I remember one time, it was so demeaning. I was sitting in the cell waiting . . . and they had a fifth grade school class coming in to see jail. That was the weirdest, the strangest feeling. I would always say to myself, "Hmm, this is such an interesting experience. Isn't my life so interesting? Now I'm getting to experience jail. Meeting all these interesting people in jail, you know like maybe someday I'll write about it, I'm just so lucky to experience this." (Laughs.) Sometimes I decided just to stay in jail. Nobody missed me. I'm like, "Oh, this one girl stabbed her boyfriend, isn't this interesting. . . . " As I started to get sober, jail wasn't much fun.

This was a more serious offense. Scott bailed me out. I was really lucky to have a rich boyfriend.

We went to court. The judge asked me questions. The lawyer was defending me, saying I was on welfare and I was in therapy. . . . The judge asked, "Well, what's the name of this therapist?" I didn't know. I couldn't answer anything. I didn't know who my therapist was. I hardly knew my name. I mean I said nothing. The lawyer said I was great. The judge gave me three years suspended sentence. He told Scott I needed to change my environment. He told him to take me up to Connecticut and things might get better.

Little did Scott know that I had been brought up there and knew people. Scott had a house in New York right on Park Avenue, and a house in Connecticut. So it was just like going home to where I started drinking. He had a huge mansion, and a huge cottage. He gave me the key to the liquor cabinet. "If you want a drink, dear . . . . " I had withdrawn from the barbiturates. I was trying not to drink. I was really trying. Scott didn't want me working because he said it didn't look right. But he never gave me any money. I felt like a prisoner there. When I got drunk I got violent, broke things, and had tantrums.

We ended up living on Scott's boat. It was there that I started experiencing this detachment from everything around me. It was as if nothing were real anymore. I felt dead all the time.

I was in therapy. Scott sent me. The therapist was supposed to be great. One day he told me he was in love with me. Scott had paid a lot of money for this, and what I was doing was letting him fuck me during our sessions. I remember leaving one of the sessions one time and looking in the rear view mirror driving back to Old Saybrook. I was laughing and crying. I looked like a mad person in my eyes, just totally mad. And there was no place to go. Except to my son.

Finally I stopped going to therapy and went to a bar instead. I told Scott why. He said, "It must have been you. You seduce them."

I felt so abandoned and so fucking shitty. I left Scott and moved into a hotel. One night I decided I was going to confront him. We had a tear-gas gun on the boat. I was drunk. I went to the boat. Scott was at a friend's house. I went to the house and I kept banging on the door. Scott came to the door. I took the tear-gas gun and held it to his face. Inside, I knew I wasn't going to do it. The neighbors didn't know if it was a real gun or not. But I really could have destroyed him. Scott didn't move. He said, "Now, dear, see how you look, blah blah blah." Some of the neighbors were out. Somebody yelled, "What kind of mother are you?"

That kind of shocked me out of it. I was looking up at the stars, thinking about Van Gogh's Starry Night. I threw the gun down. I drove about ninety miles an hour back to the hotel. The next morning Scott called. I'd thrown his engagement ring into the ocean, some family heirloom. I told him I wanted to go into a hospital. He said, "I'm glad, because as far as I'm concerned last night was attempted murder and you're either going to go into the hospital or I'm going to press charges." I was caught. But I wanted to go. I felt so detached. Everything was becoming more and more surrealistic. I wasn't attached to people anymore, not even to my own child. I knew I was gone.

So I went to a psychiatric hospital in Westport, Connecticut. I was willing. I signed the papers. He took my son. He paid cash for the hospital. He said I'd had a nervous breakdown, never mentioning my drinking or the drugs. Just "You need a rest, dear."

They didn't have detoxes then, at least not up in the North. I was in the psychiatric ward. They put me in a cage in a bed. They locked the top of the bed down. They shoot you up with Thorazine, and I was just walking around doing the thorazine shuffle. I visualized myself living there for the rest of my life scrubbing stairs. My son would come to visit someday. . . . I had this movie in my head.

They had me talk to a few psychiatrists. One guy came up to me and said he was a drug counselor. They had just put on a new wing where they were going to do a drug and alcohol program and he said, "We think that's where you belong." Thank God. He was only in this program because he was in N.A. He had no education. He was pretty much like me, a street person. His name was Tony. So I went there and they got me off the Valium. They had meetings every day. We were still locked, we still had bars on the windows. There was a woman named Judy. I'll never forget her. She was in A.A. and she was always giving me this real positive reinforcement. I'd say, "Judy, don't you know I'm violent . . . you don't understand how bad I am." She said, "You're not that bad, Mary. You're going to make it."

I stayed there for three months. I was afraid to leave. I liked it there. But still I kept saying, "I'm going to smoke pot." There was this one A.A. meeting that really hit my gut. There was a man who started talking about his insanity. We were doing the second and third step. He started talking about insanity and he started talking about the same insanity I was having. The hallucinations, the fears, the violence. It was everything I felt. I couldn't believe it. That's when I got hooked. I knew. "I'll take the first step. If giving up alcohol is going to get me out of this insanity, then I'm gonna go for it." And so I did.

I got out of the hospital. I was going to meetings. I left Scott. He said, "I paid over $6,000 for you to tell me you never loved me?" I went to Key West. I met people in the program who were smoking still, so I didn't feel too bad. This was fifteen years ago. I was thirty-four. I got into a violent relationship. I was running races, six, seven miles a day. On the outside I looked healthy, I wasn't drinking. On the inside I was still insane, still in these relationships. Not drinking, but I was totally obsessed over a guy, and his abuse was getting worse.

I began getting suicidal, realizing I was neglecting my son for this asshole. My son is probably stable because he grew up going to meetings. He knew more about the program than I ever did. From a little boy, he'd sit there on my lap. Sometimes he'd say, "Turn it over, Ma." He knew people could change. He had good teachers. I read that book, *Women Who Love Too Much*, and I identified with that. I was still waking up suicidal. I joined a Women Who Love Too Much group and the moderator didn't want anyone on drugs. Her advice to me was just to ignore this guy. Just ignore him.

I went back into A.A. where I had already received my eleventh-year medallion. I went up and took a white chip. Everyone was looking at me, "Did you drink?" And I said, "No, but I've been smoking pot all along and I just want you to know. I want to start all over again." And I joined N.A. and that was a serious move. I've been straight, clean off everything, for three years.

But I'll tell you, getting over that guy and getting off drugs are in the same category. I had to use a lot of visualization to deal with it. I would visualize myself in a swimming pool, with these guard dogs around me and if one thought of him came into my brain, these guard dogs would attack it. Whether it was good, bad, compassionate, I knew that going back to him would be going back to drugs. So I kept going to meetings.

I have the freedom today to make the decisions to change my attitude. I think before, I just went for destruction; I was not able to step back, take that leap. Now I have space between me and that. I did a lot of swimming and running. I got a grant for school. I've put a lot of energy into that and raising my son.

Now my son's leaving. He's going to go into the army and I'm going to be alone. The one difference is, I have control today. I have the ability to change. I can go to a meeting, meditate, accept my feelings. And now I have real friends. I've been off drugs, I don't feel compulsive. I don't feel paranoid anymore. Going to school has taught me to concentrate. I read more. School is difficult.

I feel good. I feel like I'm really into the spiritual part of the program. I have compassion. I can sleep a full night without a nightmare.

May 1990

Cheryl

The daughter of a salesman, and the youngest of nine children, she is thirty-six years old and works in a three-quarter house. (Some people go from a treatment center to a half-way house, to a three-quarter house where they are prepared to go back into society.) Her blonde hair is shoulder length. She has large blue eyes and a dry sense of humor. Our interview took place on the floor in a stairwell at the "house." We were interrupted every few minutes by swearing, loud voices, and alarms going off. But when she spoke she blocked the noise out and told me her story so vividly I was riveted. In the beginning she whispered but as she grew to trust me her voice became louder. The only person in charge from four P.M. to midnight, she is responsible for bed-checking and monitoring sixty recovering alcoholics. She has been sober since 1981 and lives in Boston, Massachusetts.

I'll tell you my story. My father was a heavy drinker, an alcoholic. I can remember when I was real little, just grabbing the champagne toasts off the table. I did what everyone else was doing, I was drinking. I was small, so I had to reach up onto a table to get it. I had to be pretty young, four or five. I drank what was left over, whatever I could get my hands on.

I went to a Catholic school and the nuns were real abusive. They did crazy things. Looking back now, I think I was hyperactive, and they dealt with that by taping my mouth shut and stapling my clothes to the chair. Between my father's drinking, yelling and screaming, and their abuse, I felt awful about myself. I had all this energy and I didn't know what to do with it. Alcohol killed that. It slowed me down.

I was a real scared kid. I was school-phobic. I would scream and cry because I was afraid something would happen to my mother when I went to school. I never knew what kind of condition my father would come home in. It was such a frightening thing, and I told her, "I'm never gonna get married. I'm never gonna go to school. I'm never going to go out on my own. I'm going to stay with you forever."

My father used to throw things, but he didn't hit us until the later years. He did disciplinary hitting with belts and stuff. It was emotional abuse in the early years, screaming and yelling all the time. Some of my most vivid memories are driving in the car. He would drive real fast and pass cars. I can remember peering over the dashboard. He'd play chicken with the car that was coming head on. He would veer back in line. I was terrified. Sometimes he would stop and let us get out and walk home, and sometimes he wouldn't. The verbal stuff was, "You're no good, you're nothing. You'll never be anything, you never were anything. I drink because of you." You know, "If you kids weren't such brats, I wouldn't drink."

You were drinking then?

Yeah, but only when it was around. But there were always weddings and baby showers. I was the youngest of nine kids. It was wedding after wedding, funeral after funeral, baby shower after baby shower.

By the time I was eleven I was smoking cigarettes and skipping school. I wanted out of the Catholic school. My mother let me go to public school and that was the answer. Then it wasn't the answer. I started to hang out with kids from the public school, smoking cigarettes and drinking. I skipped school and rode around in stolen cars. I really started to rebel. The anger started to come out. I used to fight a lot. It was like a pastime to get rid of my anger. I would leave my house and go look for somebody to beat up because I had all this pent-up anger and no one listened to me about anything. That's how I survived. It's how I kept my sanity. People would pick on me at home, so I'd go out and pick on somebody else.

I started hanging around with this woman and her whole family was messed up. My family, they all drank, but they had jobs and went to work and functioned—I don't know how. I started hanging around with her, and her sister got drugs for baby-sitting. It got me out of my house. I didn't have to be around my father. It was somewhere as a teen to go to get away, no one screamed at me there, or told me I was no good. I could have some peace. I was just thirteen or fourteen years old, and that's how I got into drugs. We did ups and downs and acid and speed. Finally I quit school.

I thought I'd go to work, but I couldn't function. I couldn't keep a job. As soon as I got a pay check, I just wanted to go out with my friends and get drunk, smoke pot, and walk out on all of my problems.

I went to a mental health center to a psychiatrist when I was about sixteen and told her everything that was going on. She promised not to tell my mother, but she called my mother anyway and told her everything. So I said, "I'll never go for help again." She shouldn't have lied to me. Maybe she didn't but I thought she did. Knowing me then, I used to lie so much, I might have made that up. I was so screwed up that I would embellish things to fit into my little world, that I felt so alone in.

As an adolescent I tried to talk to my mother. She would try to talk to me about my problems, but my father would scream for her to come and talk to him. He'd ask my mother if we were talking about him. She would tell him, "No, we are not." He never believed it. He would say, "I *know* you are talking about me. Now get in here and sit with me." So of course, I would be left in tears in the other room with no one to talk to. And I wanted to talk. So all the more, I started to hang around with my friend, and she had heroin. I tried it a few times. Then I got scared and got off of it.

I went to apply for welfare. A friend told me to get on mental disability, because it's more money. All you have to do is put on this big act. So I said, "Okay," and I went over and hammed it up. I didn't have too much of a problem making them believe I was crazy. I was eighteen. I went to see the psychiatrist. I was chewing these big jaw breakers and I got this red stuff all over his cards and paperwork. He said, "Go on, get out of here." He put me on mental disability with the stipulation that I stay out of my house because there was too much emotional turbulence there. I didn't tell the psychiatrist that I was drinking or doing any drugs because someone told me, "Don't tell them that because then they won't help you." So I'd said, "No way, I'm just crazy." I was scared. I was desperate.

I couldn't seem to function. I couldn't work. I couldn't go to school. I got an apartment and I did pretty good for awhile. I would go to church every morning and then I'd go to the "Y" and work out. I would have a drink with my dinner. I would say, "I will have one drink." But of course I would finish the whole bottle. You know, one drink leads to another. I would then go out to the bars, get smashed, and come home in a taxi because I was too drunk to drive or walk.

I went to the family doctor, the same one that gave my father Valium for the jitters. I told him that I was nervous, and I didn't know what was wrong with me. He said, "Here, have some Valium and don't come back." So I took them, and of course had the drink with the dinner, which led to the bars. Oh—I had come out too—I found out that I was gay. I knew all my life, but in Catholic school you don't tell anybody that. So that added to the guilt. It was just one more thing that you couldn't tell anybody about.

Did you ever have sex with a man?

Yeah, I had a boyfriend. My best friend's brother. She would always fix me up with someone so we could double date. But I was never as interested in men as I was in women.

How old were you when you had your first relationship with a woman?

Eleven. I knew before then. I knew when I was little and watched TV. I would be lusting after Marilyn Monroe instead of the guy. I knew that I'd better not tell anybody.

Why?

Well, it was normal for me, but I didn't know the name for it. I knew being brought up Catholic with the fear, the fire and brimstone, and I thought, "Oh dear, I'm doomed." It's like I'm a minority for being a woman, I'm a minority for being a lesbian. A friend of mine refers to growing up gay as ending up with the same symptoms as adult children of alcoholics. *Don't talk, don't trust, don't feel.* You're hiding all the time. It's the same stuff. I wanted to anesthetize myself, for many, many reasons. Growing up with a drinking father and a codependent mother is so. . . .

I met a woman and I fell in love. I found out she was a heroin addict. I ended up using with her. I lost the welfare check. I sold my guitar, my bike, the furniture, everything. I was not responsible enough to change my address. I was homeless. I went right back to alcohol though, after my tolerance went up from heroin. I would wake up, shoot up, drink at noon, and take pills to go to sleep.

Then I met this guy at Tony's Pizza Palace who started talking about A.A. I didn't pay too much attention. I thought he was really crazy. I said, "Oh, yeah, fine." But a couple of weeks later, I was in a bar down the street drinking at the Blue Moon Cafe, drowning my sorrows. "Woe is me, I'll never get better; this lifestyle is really disgusting." Suddenly I remembered about the A.A. meeting. I remember he'd told me they were on Saturday nights and it happened to be a Saturday night. It was right across the street in the old Alano Club, downstairs. It felt like my Higher Power had lifted me by the scruff of my shirt, off the bar stool, and walked me across the street to the meeting. The meeting was almost over and people were leaving. There was a woman there named Brenda. I started telling her everything, all these problems and she said, "Typical alcoholic thinking." She laughed. She said, "We're gonna get you to detox." And I said, "Detox? What's that?" So, there weren't any beds at detox, but she said, "I'll take you to my house, and to detox in the morning." I said, "Okay." So we went to her house and she gave me pills to go to sleep, and then alcohol in the morning and I thought, *"Who are these people?"*

I went to detox. This nurse named Sally was telling me my liver was distended. I thought she was making a big deal. I didn't believe her, and I don't remember how long I stayed there. Maybe I stayed four or five days. I went to some of their meetings and I said, "I think I need to go *in* somewhere." I said, "I want to go as far away as possible." So I went to Janus House. I stayed a month and then I ran away. It was Christmas time and I wanted to come home. I wanted to get drunk. And I did.

I went back to Janus House for four months. I got in a conflict with some women and I couldn't deal with it. I didn't know how to resolve conflicts so I ran away again. I came back here and my father was puking up his liver. I told my mother to have him go to detox and he said he'd go. I was real surprised he went.

The story I got was that he refused the medication and had a stroke. My brother said it was all my fault. I went out drinking. In A.A. meetings, they kept telling me, "It's not your fault. He would have had a stroke anyway, a worse one." But I kept hearing my brother, my big brother saying, "You're no good, you're no good, you're no good, you're bad. You did this." The same messages I'd been getting all my life.

My father went into the hospital and I went in and out of treatment centers and detox. I went to Boston, two or three Marathon houses, county detox, the Salvation Army detox, the state hospital, and Serenity House. Need I say more? I had over three hundred and fifty admissions to the Salvation Army detox.

I took my father and tried to nurse him back to health. And then somehow he got a drink. Someone gave him a drink. I don't know what happened. He went back in the hospital, and he never came back out. He got in the fetal position from fear. His legs became restricted. He died in that position.

Today I look at that, and I know that people do die from this disease. I don't want to die like that. I used to go up to visit him and read him the Big Book. I dragged him to meetings when he was still walking. He was one of the people who died, who didn't want to go to A.A. I don't know why. He didn't have the courage, or the want, to go. He didn't. He said it.

During that time I made a lot of suicide attempts. It was the only way I could ask for help. I would drink and take thirty Valiums, then I would call the hospital and ask if I should come in. I wouldn't tell 'em where I was until I was almost passed out. It was a cry for help, the only way I could ask. It was a very painful time because I knew where the help was and I wasn't accepting it. I knew where A.A. was and I wasn't accepting that. I'd go to meetings, I'd be sober for three weeks, then I'd go back out. My friends used to say, "Why do you go to all those meetings? You just come out and use again." I said, "Someday I'm gonna use what I'm learning." And they're like, "Yeah. Yeah, sure."

I really felt like I didn't want to continue drinking and drugging forever. I wanted to play as long as I could. I felt young and had time and I liked drinking. It took away the pain. Every time I put it down, I couldn't deal with all these feelings and memories from the hell I had lived.

Can you describe the pain?

I think one of the biggest reasons I had suicide attempts was because I could not accept being gay. Gay and Catholic. That was a big thing with me. A.A. was a wonderful program, but they talked about God there. The women there kept telling me it's not religion, it's spirituality. Spiritual just means yesterday I didn't want to live, and today I do. I couldn't separate religion from spirituality. I thought they wanted to get their clutches in me, and as soon as they got me around long enough they were going to tell me I couldn't be gay. The guilt that I wasn't supposed to be that way, a lesbian, was painful. I was this misfit.

You're not that way now.

Well, I've chipped away at it forever. I've let go of that old condemning God and let the new, loving God, the one that loves me— to be clean and sober for today—into my life. So the pain was about my guilt, that I should die because I'm gay. I couldn't deal with it. I knew I couldn't change it. And the world wanted me to change it. My world as I saw it. The women in A.A. kept telling me, "It's okay just who you are. That's organized religion. It has nothing to do with A.A. Not all religions are even condemning of that . . . " As soon as I started to hear that kind of stuff and look into it, I started to get more and more glimmers of hope.

I had a lover but I needed money. I was prostituting. And that was the worst part of all, of being an addict, sleeping with men and hating it. I was a junkie with a conscience. I didn't like robbing people's houses, it was terrible. I was only hurting myself this way— which I knew was bullshit. It was the lesser of two evils.

What about AIDS?

I got clean in 1981 and AIDS was just hitting New York. I would be dead if I hadn't stopped. I wouldn't be here.

I realized I had charges. I knew I was going to jail, for larceny and robbery. I was shooting $500 of coke a day. I was trying to stay sober 'cause I was pregnant. I said to my lover, "Okay, that's it." All of a sudden, I believe I had a spiritual awakening. I realized I wasn't going to get drunk because I was mad at my father, I was going to get drunk because I was an alcoholic. During all those years of A.A. I realized I was an addict, but not an alcoholic. I kept drinking trying to prove I wasn't. I was in denial, a lot of denial. When I realized that, I thought, "If this is the case, I'm gonna get good and drunk. This is going to be the last time." It was a big revelation. We went to the place where I had my first drink. It was the Blue Dolphin back then, where we'd had all our wedding receptions. Now it was a Chinese restaurant. We just drove and I said, "Pull in here." We pulled in and that was the last time I drank. Weird, because maybe that's the building where I had my first drink. My first drug was alcohol and my last drug was alcohol. It's kind of poignant, you know?

But by then I had all these charges. I was twenty-six, I was pregnant. I went back to Janus House. I said I wanted to come back. I told them I was pregnant. Here I am, I'm gay and pregnant. I thought they'd say, Here she comes with one of her "yets."* Because that's exactly how I saw it; one more awful thing that I had no control over. But they said come anyway.

I didn't go to jail. They gave me a couple years' probation and suspended everything. Then, four months sober, my baby was born. They said he's okay, and then at three in the morning they said he's in withdrawal. I was four months clean and I said, "I don't understand how this can be." They said he lost oxygen somewhere along the line in the birthing process. During the labor I was okay, 'til this doctor—I had a midwife and I shouldn't have done that. I was a high-risk pregnancy and the midwife couldn't deliver because I never dilated—this doctor, who everyone's suing, which I found out later, comes out of nowhere, and says, "How do you feel about a cesarean?" I said, "I don't know." He said, "I have a meeting to go to, I'll be back in two hours." That's when I lost it. I started screaming. Before that, I was saying the serenity prayer, doing breathing exercises. I had gone to a childbirth class. I mean, when I got clean I

*An A.A. term for not yet, or "yet" to happen.

was a totally different person. So the doctor left and I started screaming, "Get him back."

They knew my baby was in distress. The doctor should have taken
the baby right then and there but he didn't. Two hours later they
took me in and did a cesarean. Then at three in the morning they
said he was in withdrawal and he had seizures, and had lost oxygen.
They came in and told me the next day that everything was fine.
That was a lie.

I didn't find out until he was six months old that he'd lost oxygen.
And it was severe. He has cerebral palsy. He's multi-handicapped,
legally blind and he has seizures. He's on medication for the seizures.
He was in an incubator and they were putting phenobarbital in him
to stop the seizures. I was doing $500 of coke a day, and drinking.
So I've done a lot of work on the guilt, and I tried to sue the doctor.
Later, the midwife told me the meeting was about whether I was
really clean and sober or not. My prenatal care was perfect, but they
said "You can't believe 'em." Meaning addicts and alcoholics. I was
honest, about what I took, to protect the baby. It's ironic. So ge-
netically he's hyperactive, I'll cop to that. Sleep disturbances, I'll cop
to that. But the loss of oxygen, I believe, is their fault. And yes, I've
dealt with a lot of guilt. It's been hard. He's eight and he's super.
His name is Mark. I stayed sober. I took him to a handicapped play
group, learned everything I could, sat and worked with him and
took him to Healing Mass.

At church I thought, "If they knew I was gay would they support
me?" No. I brought the priest a plate of cookies me and my lover
baked, and he never even thanked us. It was like ever since I started
bringing her, he was snubbing me. There came a time when I had
one foot in A.A. and one foot in the Catholic Church. I had to put
them both somewhere, so I put them in A.A.

How do you feel about men now?

There are a lot of healing men. I've looked for them, and it's trial
and error. Sometimes I think, he's a healing person, a healing man,
but I get close and he's not; he turns out to be abusive and then I
say, "That's unfortunate." I had a lot of hurts from men in my life
and I needed to be healed. Even though I don't have them in my life
the way straight women do, I have them as friends.

How do you feel about being a woman in A.A.?

A.A. is just a composite of the world. I'm going to like some people and I'm not going to like other people. Some people are real sick and some people are healthier. I can learn from the healthier ones. I can also learn from the sick ones. My father died from alcoholism and I stayed sober. My lover that I started shooting dope with crashed on the highway drunk when I was two and a half years sober. She was drunk. She died. That really hurt a lot.

And you didn't relapse?

No. Well, I already had all those relapses in and out for seven years. I pray to them, I say, "I'm still here trying to do this, your struggle's over. If you can send me some strength please do 'cause this is hard." Day in, day out, dealing with feelings and not taking something to cover the pain. Learning, for the first time in my life, how to deal with problems and conflicts, the hum-drumness after I lived this exciting life before. I mean there's times when I miss hanging off fire-escapes, kicking cans, drinking beers, and spitting. That's my vision of "no responsibility" and that's what I ran from was responsibilities. I wanted an easier, softer way. I wanted to be rich, but I didn't want to work for any of it. I didn't think I should have to, after the stuff I put up with as a kid.

What would you say to a woman struggling with alcoholism?

Don't give up. No matter how many times you fall, you get up, dust yourself off, and you try again. You will make it if you don't give up.

In the beginning I couldn't even go to gay meetings, I was so homophobic. Some gay people don't want to go to straight meetings but my advice is, "Venture out, go to some straight meetings too."

Being sober and clean is not being afraid anymore to stand up for your rights and walk—walk and not be afraid to walk where you want to walk. A.A. is free therapy and that's where you take risks, and you reach out to certain people and when they don't reach back, or shun you—*if you don't take risks you won't grow, you won't grow up. You stop growing emotionally when you start drinking.* So when people put it down, they're like thirteen years old. And they're whining. They just have to learn that they can't have their way all the time, and they have to grow up, find their niche, learning all the way.

I jumped into another relationship with a woman who's recovering. I'm really codependent. I went back to school, and I'm in a substance abuse counseling certification program, which is a two-year degree program. After I went back to school I was beginning to blossom and my lover felt threatened, and I'm like, "What is this crap?" So I left, and all summer I dated. Recently I went back again. It's better, better than ever. I conquered my fear of living alone. Al-Anon is what helped me, 'cause we were gonna kill each other fighting. I was going to go into treatment for codependency if this didn't work, but it did.

I think I'm sober because I go to three to five meetings a week. I don't just go to meetings, I raise my hand and talk about what's going on. I take that risk, and I dump the garbage. I know that I would not be here otherwise. I know that alcoholics isolate their feelings, and that's where it begins. When people start drinking again, it's because they begin to isolate. They stop sharing at meetings. Eventually, they stop going to meetings, and that's it, they start using. So the big thing is, continue to share at your meetings. Try to raise your hand at every meeting, and talk, *talk about what is going on with you.* I was taught growing up, "Don't talk about your problems, don't tell the neighbors." But if I don't tell everyone my business now, I will die. I have to tell because *we're as sick as our secrets.* I will get sick again if I don't share. So I dump it, and miraculously, I feel better.

April 1990

Part Three

Identity: Searching for a Voice

When those we devastate and crush are
finally lost and driven away and are perished
in the danger. for then I want In the rubble
heaps at last to hear my voice again, which
was a howling from the very first.

—Rainer Maria Rilke,
translated by Edward Snow

Liz

Fifty-seven and divorced, Liz is a counselor for a small treatment center in New England. Her father and ex-husband are doctors. She graduated from a distinguished college for women in New England, and recently applied to graduate school for her master's in social work. Parts of her story were taken from an autobiographical sketch she wrote as part of the entrance requirement. She is beautiful in a classic sense. Her high cheekbones, delicate nose, and cap of straight brown hair give her an air of distinction. Her blue eyes welcomed me. At once I noticed two qualities about her that complement one another: thoughtfulness and self-assertion. She dislikes pretension, but is not blind to human frailty; when people in treatment centers disguise themselves to appear fragile she sees through the pose. She enforces honesty in herself but takes care with the feelings of others. I imagine that in the presence of a manipulative patient she sees also a person in pain. For Liz, Alcoholics Anonymous is more than a means to sobriety. It is a place where she feels comfortable, relaxed. She found her way there in 1982 and has been sober since that time. She lives in Vermont and has four grown daughters.

"I was born in 1932," she writes in her autobiography, "to a family of professional men and their college-educated wives. I am the eldest of four daughters, and a college education was both promised and expected. The unspoken message was that you go to college to become an interesting person—interesting to whom was left unexplained. Gradually it became clear that girls got married and had babies and that this made it very, very difficult to be a doctor, though some women did it. The implication was that these women usually failed at some aspect of child care and were vaguely selfish or not dedicated to their marriages.

"Graduation in 1954 revealed a powerful need to make a plan. I enrolled in a six-week secretarial course in Cambridge, Massachusetts, in order to get a job. At a "mixer" I met six young men and they all called. My social life became complicated and absorbing. Very soon one relationship singled itself out; in the space of one year I was engaged to marry a medical student in his third year. We were married in September of 1955.

"We moved through the training process for physicians. Fort Bragg, North Carolina; Baltimore; Lexington, Kentucky; Ann Arbor, Michigan; and in 1967, we arrived in upstate New York."

When did you start drinking?

The longer I'm sober the more I realize it was earlier than I had first thought. I'd say somewhere in my twenties. I discovered that if I drank I was more comfortable, I wasn't so anxious or fearful. Then I realized that if I was tense or sad or even very happy, I drank to take the edge off, in order to maintain an even social state. In my family you didn't express a lot of emotions. Happiness was one thing but no sort of anxiety or pain was acceptable. "Go to your room until you feel better." I found out that all that emotion was easier to take care of after having a drink.

When I married and things got tense between me and my husband, I'd have a drink. This was all very once-a-weekish for quite a long time, I'd say 'til about the mid-sixties, when it began to be more than once a week. It began to be every night. Finally, it got to be I didn't want there *not* to be any booze in the house, whether or not I drank it. But I always drank it.

In the mid-seventies the marriage started going bad. By going bad I mean that I was not able emotionally or sexually to deal with stress, or disapproval or correction or "I can't stand this," or "I want you to do that." I would always do what I was told to do and wouldn't even know that I didn't like it for the longest time. If I didn't like it there was something the matter with *me*, not anything the matter with what I was being asked to do. So I would have a drink.

When he decided to leave I really started to drink. He didn't want to be home with us. He was uncomfortable, he would say he was uncomfortable. After a while he began going away by himself and I would stay with the kids and the next step was for him to find other company. The next step was for him to leave for good. We were divorced in 1976.

Then I drank even more; I had an excuse—poor me. I had to go to work. I went back to work and got into very contentious situations, such as being the new secretary in the physics department, and getting yelled at. I couldn't handle it at all. Plus the girls were sixteen, fifteen, twelve, and eight and they would give me flack about their hours, boyfriends or activities. So I drank, which I thought was really appropriate, rather than spend a lot of money on shrinks.

We were really short on money because the alimony and child support wouldn't be enough and I'd have to ask my family to help or just do without. Or the children would do without and I'd tell them, "It's Dad's fault." He would come pick them up with a new car and they would yell at him for having a new car. "How come we don't even have our sport jackets?" Some of the things they wanted were appropriate. Some of it was just being adolescent. I couldn't make any sense out of what was appropriate and what wasn't. I would just do the best I could but I'd get polluted in the evening. It was a bad time for everyone, but in spite of it all the girls qualified for college entrance. At that time I didn't know about the children of alcoholic parents—their need to excel and prop up family appearances, support the ailing parent.

What were you drinking?

I was drinking whatever there was. Usually vodka, or sherry. At first it was just sherry. Then sherry in a glass but vodka added, to make it stronger. Then I could limit myself to so and so many drinks.

What did it feel like to sit down with a drink?

I thought of it as peace. This is my medication. Now I can handle whatever I need to do. At first I just sipped it, but later on, just before I stopped, I'd be knocking back a couple just to take the edge off. Then, if I had to drive anywhere, I wasn't even slightly drunk. That was just bringing me up to a normal level. My tolerance was such that I could handle quite a lot. Two drinks in and I felt fine, just normal. I was making dinner—I thought—but of course now the girls tell me I was always making the same thing. I always made omelettes and they can't look at an omelette now. If I drove to pick them up, I'd have trouble finding where they were; they'd have to wait.

I began to have anxiety attacks. I began to have anxiety, real high anxiety, and thought that it had to do with my being alone, so I'd drink more to take care of the anxiety and the anxiety got worse. Liquor works fast. Bingo. It's a central nervous system depressant. I didn't know panic was one of the symptoms of withdrawal or a part of the alcoholism.

Your anxiety attacks were alcohol induced?

Pretty much. It certainly didn't help. I probably would have been highly anxious whether I was drinking or not. I'm still anxious, but I haven't had an anxiety attack in a while. I get them when I don't know how to cope. I had one a year ago—not quite a full-blown one—but I had a lot of anxiety at my mother's decline. It was due to her moving out of her house and moving into a retirement community. She put me down around my fears of being old. She would give me a hard time and I would feel fear. I've had anxiety attacks since I quit drinking, but not to the same extent.

I got stopped by the police one night around 1977. I'd been drinking. I put a peppermint in my mouth before I left the house because I had gotten an unexpected phone call to go pick up Emma at the high school after swimming. I went through a yellow light. I went to the side of the road and a little bit off the road, and came back on. At the next turn, a cop stopped me and told me I had gone through a red light and off the road. I said, "I know I went through the yellow, but I was going too fast to stop." I tried to talk myself out of it. I told him about my daughter with the wet hair, but I was really embarrassed. I was humiliated, and I thought, "Oh shit." Emma was waiting at the high school and the idea of explaining what happened . . . I thought he was going to give me a DWI but he didn't. He let me go, but that was a big significant factor, a red flag.

I began blacking out in the late evening when the kids would call me. I had strict rules about them calling me if they were going to be late. They would call and I'd forget they'd called or they would tell me they'd be home in an hour and I would jump all over them when they came home, because I didn't remember. I'd forget which kid it was who had called if two or three would be out. I'd be drinking, falling asleep, and I couldn't remember who had called and who hadn't, so there was a lot of inappropriate scolding. And they would play little games with me too. They got smart, plus they were drinking themselves. Deb still scolds me for not recognizing that she was drinking up a storm in high school. I kind of knew it, but I didn't know what to do about it. My opinion *still* is there wasn't a whole lot I would've been able to do about her drinking. But of course she's right. I should have said something. It would have been good to have recognized how much she was drinking.

Another thing happened that was embarrassing, I said I would help with this local candidate for city council, calling people and stuff like that. He had a meeting of all the workers and I went there drunk. I was late and he, as a nice guy gesture, had me come up and sit with him, facing all the other workers. I know I just stank of alcohol. I must have, and that embarrasses me—plus a couple of phone calls I can remember—and I'm sure there were others. Deb has some beauts that she tells me about, but I've only just felt ready to hear them because I have a tremendous amount of guilt about all that, still. I felt like I should have done it perfectly. I should have been perfect. I should have not . . . done this, whatever it was that they had noticed or would report to me. That's codependency—meaning what the other person sees in you, thinks of you, or observes is the most important thing; not what you yourself think, observe, or see as important.

In April 1982 I was mixed up in a relationship that I wanted to end. The relationship had a lot to do with drinking, not on his part, but on mine. He would drink too—but he wouldn't get drunk. He couldn't begin to drink as much as I could. He was a very nice man who was needy, who needed a woman. He's a minister and he really needed a wife. He thought I'd make a good candidate. He would take me out and we'd drink and talk and get all theological and philosophical. The more I drank the more philosophical I'd get. I couldn't remember a thing afterwards, not one thing. I couldn't remember all these big points I'd be making. I knew it wasn't going to work. I wanted to get out of it and felt guilty so I just hitched it right onto the drinking. I said, "This relationship is based on alcohol, so I have to stop it." Just completely fallacious. His side wasn't based on alcohol but mine was, big time. Every time we stopped drinking it was just—yawn. He was very bright too, very earnest, really a decent person. I was screwing around with it, so it's good that I got out of it. He, I think, was more into it than I was; that was unfair. Plus he was a friend of a very good friend of mine from college and that's how we met each other. I don't think they think too much of me now. It was all kind of icky.

In 1981 Linda came back from the Peace Corps. She told me I was drinking a whole lot more than when she'd left. She'd been away for two years. That was a clear demarcation for her. She was going to go to graduate school and wanted to come home and live cheap until she went. She'd noticed there was an awful lot of booze going down and told me so. I told her to go to hell, to mind her own business, and if she didn't like what was going on in my house she could find another place to stay. She stopped telling me about it for a couple of months; then she told me again. She said she was going to take Emma, the youngest, with her to a mental health association which was giving a three-night seminar, a couple of hours each, for the children of alcoholics. I said, "Like hell!" She planned this and it was coming up. I got on the phone and called a local agency for evaluation assessment and group therapy. I got into a group with a facilitator and nobody even asked me about my alcoholism; it was a given. The first night I said nothing. By the second night, I was known as an alcoholic. I wasn't going to go to A.A. because that was for "those people," the ones with long raincoats and the little bottles in brown bags. About three or four other people in the group said they weren't going to go to A.A. either because that was for the people in the raincoats with the brown paper bags and bottles. Then they laughed. Pretty soon I was laughing too.

The only way to stay in the group was to go to one A.A. meeting a week and you couldn't cheat. There was a very attractive, intelligent woman in the group who said, behind her hand as I walked out of the meeting, "If you ever want to talk to a drunk lady, give me a call." I said, "Okay," but I vowed never to call her because I had to be perfect. After a year of sobriety, I did call her. She talked me into going to Hazelden, a treatment center, for thirty days.

So I *did* go to the A.A. meeting because that was required. Then they had me pick up this kid who didn't have a car because of DWI trouble, and take him to the group. That hit all my responsibility buttons. So I picked him up and that got me there. That's how I got to A.A.

Then I came to like A.A. a lot. I felt right at home. It was a welcoming type group. In A.A. I met people I never would have met otherwise: doctors' wives, physicists' wives. My boss's wife tottered in briefly before she committed suicide.

What would you tell a woman who was having problems with A.A.?

Don't drink and go *do* something. Go to an agency where there are lists of other therapeutic groups. I would try to make sure she wasn't isolating. I'm talking more or less like a counselor because I know what's out there. If I was only familiar with A.A. I might have trouble, but there are other forms of counseling.

You can make arrangements based on your ability to pay. I'd make sure, also, that she wasn't all by herself, white-knuckling her sobriety. It depends on the woman. Usually if someone hits enough A.A. meetings, her story is going to come out and she's going to be able to relate to someone.

You love A.A.

Yes, because it's a place to go and talk where people understand. Other people don't understand. Some of them do, but I don't want to talk about the things that terrify me, or the behavior of my children, or what my ex is threatening me with, or my reaction to what my ex is. If it's about divorce, you can find any number of people in or out of the program who want to talk about the bastards and what they're up to. I would get an audience, but not a way to do something about it. At A.A. you can find a way to let it go, to deal with what needs to be dealt with day by day, to figure out what you can do, make a list, then do those things. Then ask for the ability to let it go until the next time. For example: bill paying. I had a huge stack of bills and very little money. The whole concept was, "If I pay that bill I won't have any money." Then of course a few drinks didn't hurt at all on that one. . . . So I wouldn't pay any bills, because

I was fearful that if I paid those bills there would be a drain. That's the self-defeating behavior you can get yourself into. "If I don't fix the car I won't have to pay for it." Right. So then the car just stops in the middle of nowhere and you've got to pay four or five times as much. People in A.A. would sit me down and say, "Okay, is there anyone you can borrow money from?" Yes. So I'd make a phone call, borrow money and pay my bills. But before I could do that I needed for people to say, "What can you do about this today?" That gets rid of a lot of free-floating crap.

"Just for today" helped me a lot because I was into the future all the time. If I don't do this, then that terrible thing will happen. Then I'd do something really strange, sort of a preventive voodoo type of thinking, all kinds of crazy stuff like wearing a certain dress or certain clothes. "Don't ever miss work!"—that's really common with alcoholics. "Always be on time at work or else," you could get reported—your credit will then plummet. My credit rating was already in the basement, mind you. Unknown worse things would happen to you. I would be at work while my kids were doing all the housework, making all the meals, doing most of the shopping, taking care of themselves and taking care of their little sisters.

Did you blame them for your drinking?

No, not outwardly. I would say I needed a drink for all this anxiety because they were out late, but most of the time they were in when they said they would be. They would take the credit cards and shop but they never ran over the limit. A couple of them were just so frozen with the same anxiety I had that they wouldn't buy anything. "I don't need it, Ma, I don't need it, we need the money for something else." They were very supportive, "Don't worry. We won't spend too much money. We'll take care of everything."

*How do you feel when people in treatment don't get coins?**

That's a blow. It's a blow because the coin becomes too important. It's a symbol of completing treatment successfully and there are

---

* *A coin is given to model patients after they complete treatment.*

plenty of counselors who say, "Look, it's a clinical tool." As a case manager you need to access the pain of not getting a coin. You really have to think of the effect of not getting the coin as much as the effect of getting a coin. So I normally give coins. It's very difficult to decide who's going to stay sober and who's not. A lot of coin people get drunk on the way home. A lot of non-coin people stay sober. A good friend of mine didn't get a coin. She went to Hazelden. But she refused to go to a half-way house and she refused to go to the aftercare they set up for her in Boston. She knew that the place where they were going to send her was a sleazy place in a dangerous neighborhood. So she didn't get a coin. She was crushed. But she stayed sober.

If a woman is sober and happy, say outside of A.A., isn't that the bottom line?

Yes, although I'd say it's a loss. There's so much support and fun in A.A.—opportunities to do things sober. I'm just glad it's there. That's where I found people who understood what I was talking about. When I was talking about fear, fear of what I was doing or saying, acting on another person—they all knew what I was saying. I didn't even have to finish a sentence. If I talked about that in PTA, or over coffee with one of my solid friends, they would give me advice. They would ask, "How long has it been since you've slept with somebody?" Or, "I could introduce you to this wonderful Jewish man." I did that a few times because I had a fantasy that Jewish people were more caring.

How would you help a woman who was drinking?

I'd ask how many problems have you had with drinking? Can you identify the effects of your drinking that you don't like, or that others have presented you with? Pain, what is the pain of your drinking? Then if she told me, probably by that time she'd be crying, telling me about all these things. If she said, "But I *can't* stop, but I'm *afraid* to stop, it gives me this relief," I'd say, "Go to A.A. Don't take a drink tonight, go to a meeting instead." I'd point out a meeting I thought would be really good. I'd say, "I'm going and I'd like to see you there. Let's go. We can have coffee." It would be ideal if there was a really solid women's group. You've got to remember that your job is to bring the message. Once we get sober we immediately want to make everyone else sober, using our system. Then if we feel that person is being resistant, hostile, antagonistic, we're back into that, "It's because I didn't say the right thing." So it's like, wait a second, it's not in my hands. I bring the message. My job isn't to make anyone else sober. It's about letting go of control, letting them do what they have to do.

In the Big Book, Bill outlines, "Get 'em while they're hungover, because people usually call when they're drunk." I say, "I think you're drinking, I want to hear from you tomorrow." That's what I do. I don't talk to people when they're drunk, not anymore.

You're not using A.A. slogans, you're saying some of the same things, but you're saying them in your own words.

I've worked at it. Plus I'm in the field. You can't just do slogans because they're so broad. They're valuable because they cover a lot of territory, but don't mean a whole lot unless the person gives you her specifics.

Did you love being drunk, aside from relieving the anxiety? Did you also love the high?

Oh, yes. But it didn't always come. Near the end it stopped coming altogether.

January 1990

Sylvia

A large woman in her mid-forties, Sylvia grew up in Manhattan. She went through Conifer Park, a treatment center in New York. When I asked her about her experience as a black woman in recovery she said, "I think we have a harder time than white people do. We don't like to admit to having this disease. It's a pride issue." Single and residing in Springfield, Massachusetts, she works as a sales clerk in a toy store. Both of her parents were alcoholics. We met at an Alcoholics Anonymous meeting. She has been sober since 1986.

I was really drinking from day one. My father used to give us little sips out of his drink. My mother told me that whenever they had company, no matter what time, seeing that my mother and father's door was closed, I would get up, go around and drain all the bottles and beer cans and glasses. I would walk around dizzy and lopsided and giggling. I was only three or four years old.

When I was eleven years old my mother and father were on the verge of breaking up. We were the kind of normal family where you never see the mother and father argue. Unbeknownst to us children, they did a fair share of arguing and fighting. They always did it when we were asleep.

One night they got to fighting and it woke us all up: my sister, my brother and me. That's how bad it was. My sister and my brother were throwing beer cans at my father to try and get him off my mother. It was new to us. We'd never seen them fight. Finally they stopped. My mother got my sister and brother to bed and I was sitting at the kitchen table. She came into the kitchen. She sat with me and she kept saying, "Sylvia, go on to bed." I could tell that if I lay down and went to sleep, she wouldn't be there when I got up. She kept telling me, "Oh, no, no, no, don't worry, I'll be here, da, da, da." Like they say, out of the mouths of babes? For some reason, I knew.

I must've fallen asleep at the table because the next thing I knew, I was waking up on the bed and my father was asking me, "Who do you want to live with, me or your mother?" Now, how do you ask three children that never saw their mother and father argue, and never knew there was any type of problem, who you want to live with? We didn't know how to choose.

We ended up staying with my father. From that point on my father always kept liquor in the house and I used to steal his beer and drink it until I got sleepy, then go to bed.

At eleven years old I had to do what you call "grow up." There was no more running outside with my friends. I had to be the one to cook, clean, to make sure my sister's hair was done as well as my own hair. I had to take over where my mother left off.

I'd get up in the morning, and get the three of us ready for school. I'd have to make sure we all had breakfast. Make sure my father's lunch was ready for him to take to work. Go to school, come home, clean up, iron, do everything that my mother used to do for us.

Where did she go?

The night she left, that morning or whatever, she went to her mother's house. My grandmother was not at home and, in getting out of the house, she had forgotten her set of keys. My mother used to say that she believed if my grandmother had been home that night, to let her in the house, she would come back with us. But by her mother not being home, she ended up married to another man.

It had to be at least a year until we saw her again. I remember I was twelve years old.

Did you miss her?

Yeah. A lot. Because I guess, like most people, I blamed myself. Maybe if I'd of been a better daughter she wouldn't have left. Maybe if me and my sister and brother had did what we were supposed to, like we was *told* to do, her and my father wouldn't have fought, wouldn't have broken up. So there was a lot of guilt: maybe it was my fault.

She always said it had nothing to do with me, my sister and my brother. She loved us, right? But she could no longer live with my father. Then I began to feel the resentment because I couldn't understand why she didn't take us with her. Everybody else whose mother left their father, or vice versa, they were always with their mother. Why did we have to be with my father? Not that we loved my father any less than my mother, but I guess it's just, the mother is the one. . . . She explained that she had nowhere to take us. If she'd of took us that night, with my grandmother not being there, where would we have slept? When I started getting sober, I started understanding where my mother was coming from.

Before I got sober I blamed my mother for a lot of the stuff that was wrong with me. If she'd of been a better parent, if she'd of did what she was supposed to do, I wouldn't have turned out the way I was.

I was fifteen years old and I got drunk. I was at some friends' house, boys that you're raised up with, you know. I'm waiting for the mother to come in and those two boys raped me. Threatened me that if I ever told anybody, what they were going to do to me. I probably never would've told anybody about it but the next morning my cousin Geneva had came up from downtown. I was scared to go to bed. I fell asleep on the couch. There was blood everywhere. She asked me what happened and I told her, "If I tell you, you got to promise not to tell nobody, not even daddy." And she said, "I won't tell." When I went on to tell her what was what, she said, "Okay, I'll be right back," and she went down the hall to a neighbor's house so she could use the phone to call my father.

Next thing I knew my father and his girlfriend were coming through the door. They took me to the hospital and the doctor said that they had ripped me but it was from me being scared that I bled so much. I'll never forget the doctor looking at me and saying, "Well, I hope this doesn't change your attitude toward men." I didn't know what he was talking about. I said, "What do you mean?" He said, "Well, you know most women, when a trauma like this happens to them at such a young age, they don't want anything to do with men again, all they want to have is . . . they deal with their own sex then."

So I turned around and I said, "You know what?" I says, "Maybe it's from something my mother taught me a long time ago, or something my father said, but just because one or two people did something to me, that doesn't make everybody bad." I said, "So I have to deal with it myself." I never went into therapy for that, but I should have, because I believe to this day now, that until I was about seventeen, I was always built up older. I looked like I was about nineteen or twenty in the body. But in the face, you knew I was a young kid. If you took the time to look.

Did you start building up a resentment towards men because of that incident?

I know I've never trusted men since then. I tried, you know, don't get me wrong, I've lived with three men in my life, but I never really got involved. I was living with them and doing what was expected of a wife. But it was never really all of me. It felt like I was on the outside watching what was going on. I believe subconsciously this is why I started putting on weight. I said to a friend, "Maybe I should have gotten counseling at the time." "Sylvia," she says, "it's not too late to get counseling." But it was so long ago, you know. What can they do that's going to make me feel any different about it? So like I said, I started putting on weight and I didn't take it off. I turned around and I said, "Well, I'm going on a diet." I started losing weight. I would lose weight to the point that if a fella turned around and said, "Hey, babe, you lookin' good," that was the end of the diet. I stopped right away. Because there's a fear there now if I get small something's going to happen. So I don't even deal with that no more. I'm comfortable with the way I am now. I guess not completely, because otherwise I wouldn't even talk about it. As far as having a resentment against men, I don't think it's a resentment, I think it's a natural fear that they're going to hurt me again.

I got drunk after that happened. I had gone to the community center for a dance that they had for the kids. I had met up with some other friends and we started drinking. We were drinking vodka and we were laughing. Whoever we could get to go to the store, whatever they brought back, we drank. So by the time my cousin got there I was flying. My cousin turned around and she said, "Well, Sylvia, you're already feeling good, so me and Patty, we have to turn around and try and get nice." So she said, "Come on, we're going to try and get somebody to go in the liquor store and get us a couple of bottles of wine." They always took me with them because I had no problem, like I said I was built up. We got two fifths of Thunderbird and we went across the street from the community center into this building, second floor, like in between the staircase, and we sat there and drank these two fifths of wine. I do not remember getting back to the community center. Finally, what I remember about the experience is going to my aunt's bed, laying down on the bed, the whole bed lifting up and spinning and all I can think of is, "Dear God, if you let me get over this, I will never drink no Thunderbird again." Do you know, in all my years of drinking since then, the only thing they could not get me to drink was Thunderbird. After that I didn't touch anything to drink until I was seventeen. Then, being with different people, I would drink like one or two drinks. If I started feeling it, I wouldn't touch no more, because I was too scared if I lay down, the bed was going to spin again.

At eighteen, I got introduced to marijuana. The more I tried to do, the worse my life got, so, hey, I'll go on and I'll party. I'll have a good time, and I won't worry about nothing as long as I pay my rent and I know when I get home there's someplace for me to lay down. I have no children, so why do I have to worry about spending my money?

When my brother and my cousin moved in is when I really got into smoking marijuana because we had three paydays in the house. There was never a time when you didn't come to our house and couldn't get some herb or wine. They used to call me the hoarder because they would buy it, and, you know those little film cases? I would have three or four of them. They'd bring the ounce in and I'd go and fill up one or two of them and bring them in my room because they're going to be looking for some, and hey, I got it all, you know. So I got into herb that way.

I started working for the government in '76 and met a girlfriend of mine. We used to spend weekends together, and we'd just sit there and party and get high and listen to the music. One particular night, she had some Seconols. She knew that if you took a Seconol and you drank beer with it, you could feel nice. So we drank beer and we took these Seconols. We were partying and what not and all of a sudden everything went black. I don't remember nothing until we woke up the next morning and I was like, "When did so-and-so leave?" She didn't even know. We had both passed out from it. Unbeknownst to me, I was suffering from blackout drinking. At that time, I blamed it on the pills, you understand what I'm saying? And I said, no, well, I'm not taking Seconols no more because they make me black out. I tried LSD. I didn't like that because I don't like bad trips. All it takes is one time to go bad for me and I don't want to deal with it no more.

I remember the first and only time I ever tried Methadone. Methadone used to come in a biscuit that was quartered; you could break it into quarters if need be. But we never tried it before. The fellow who was giving it to me, he took one of the quarters and cut that in half and stuck it in about two inches of water and I drank that down and then he gave me a beer behind that. I remember feeling good from it and everything was fine and it was like, ohh, I *like* it. I don't remember if I went to sleep that night, but I got dressed for work the next morning and I felt really good all day. All of a sudden I started coming down from that Methadone. I started nodding, you know, how the junkies do. I didn't like that because I was at work. Now maybe if I'd of been home, it would have been a different story, but here I am at work, I have to deal with the public. What would it look like for them to come by and I'm nodding out on them?

In '87, I got arrested for smoking cocaine. We used to buy it and I loved how the high came. I could cook it with the best of them. When it got to the point where I was buying my stuff, not letting no one know I had it, going in my house and locking my door, there was something in me saying, "Sylvia, you need help," but I didn't listen to it. In January of '87, I tried to commit suicide for the first time.

I don't know why. It wasn't like a conscious thought came on me like bam, kill yourself. I was high. I had been smoking a pipe and I'll never forget it. There was my girlfriend, Carla, and another fella. They were at my house and we had just finished smoking and we were sitting there laughing and talking. She said that all of a sudden I started crying. She said she watched me go in the closet. I'd come out of the closet and go in the bathroom. I'd be in the bathroom a few minutes, come out of the bathroom, sit down, then I would get up and go in the closet again. The routine kept going until I got up and went in the closet the last time, and then went into the bathroom. She turned around and walked in the closet 'cause she couldn't understand what was in the closet. Then she saw all the empty pill bottles.

She called the cops who in turn called an ambulance. I refused to give them any information concerning me; I just wanted to leave. I kept saying I was a burden on my mother.

They got me to the hospital. The only thing I can remember about the first six days there was they asked me, "Are you pregnant?" and I said, "Not that I know of," which, as far as I knew, I wasn't, right? The first five days they said I was in a coma. When I did come out of it, I remember this woman; she said that I should sign myself onto the psychiatric ward. She said it would only be for a week to ten days, to try and get help with a doctor. I was all for it because I knew I needed help. Anytime you try and hurt yourself, there's something wrong. I told her okay and I remember they more or less left me alone and let me sleep for three days. There were group therapy sessions where they try to get you to talk and I kept telling the doctors I wanted some kind of help. I said, "I smoke cocaine, I snort cocaine, I smoke reefer, I drink, I need some kind of help, I want to stop." They turned around and told me they would give me the help I needed, blah, blah, blah. Then I remember bugging them about, "Well, will I be out in time for my birthday?" They said, "Yeah, you'll be out in time for your birthday," which was January 22, 1987. They let me out the day before my birthday.

I had money from when I went into the hospital. I must've had about one hundred and fifty dollars on me because I had gotten my welfare check. I had all my money with me. I was on my way up the stairs and my girlfriend, the same friend who had called the hospital and everything, she was coming down the stairs. I asked her, "Where you going?" She said, "I'm going to pick up a kit." And I said, "Well, come on into the house with me and I'll give you some money to pick up some for me." Two days after getting out of the hospital, I was right back to doing what I had been doing before.

My family hadn't heard from me in two years. When I got to doing drugs I didn't want anybody in my family to see me. So it was like I dropped off the face of the earth. I cut my phone off. If they sent letters to try and get in touch with me, I wouldn't answer them. So they didn't know whether I was alive or dead. March the 3rd, 1987, exactly six weeks after the first episode, I tried to commit suicide for the second time. This time when the cops came, they searched my house until they found something with a phone number on it, which was an invitation that my mother had sent me for her seventy-fifth birthday, which I took and threw in a drawer. They found it and they called my mother.

When I looked up, my mother and my sister and my baby brother were coming through the emergency room, because they have an emergency room when they're going to send you up to the psych ward. There was nothing I could say about it then. They had to send me there because this was the second time I had tried to do that. I cried with my mother. My mother had noted that my hair was matted. I had stopped taking care of myself. The clothes I had on were the pits. I told my mother I wanted help. I told my oldest brother I wanted help. I determined I had to get some kind of help, because I told them if I had to come back there one more time, they might as well bury me because I wouldn't live through a third time inside a psych ward. My brother asked me, "Are you sure you want the help?" I said, "Yes, I want the help, I want to live." My brother got me into Conifer Park. I turned around and I said, "What about my cat?" My mother said, "You can always get another cat." I had nothing. All the clothes I had were the ones I had at the hospital.

My mother took them. I'm thinking she's going to take them to her house and wash them out, but she threw them out. When I came out of the hospital, I only had the clothes on my back, which were clothes that she had bought for me to come home in. My mother's sister, she bought me two outfits. My family started helping me because they saw that I really wanted some kind of help. My brother called and gave me the telephone number for Conifer Park. I called them, they gave me a long list over the phone of what I could bring and what I couldn't bring. They wanted to come and get me the next morning, but the stuff that they wanted me to have, I no longer had it.

I called my mother on her job that day and when she came home that night she took me shopping to make sure that I had everything that I needed to go to this treatment center.

What is it in you that makes us want to go into a treatment center with the nicest things?

I really don't know. Maybe it's because you don't want nobody to think you're as bad as everybody thinks you are. Anyway, we had to go to A.A. meetings every night. We had to go to classes every day; group therapy every day. We had one-on-one therapy every day, you know, all kinds of things. I was there a week and this particular Saturday they were showing us this film about addiction to cocaine, showing those of us who were addicted to cocaine the way I was with smoking, how it was psychological. All of a sudden I got real cold and then I started shaking and couldn't stop shaking. They took my blood pressure, took my temperature, nothing was wrong with me. The floor monitor wanted me to go ahead and lie down and I told her point blank, how scared I was. I had never talked to her like that before. I told her, if I lay down that I wouldn't wake up. She asked me why was I feeling like that and I told her I didn't know, but I knew if I lay on that bed when she told me to, that I was going to die. So they let me sit up all night and eventually it eased. It was a feeling I never want to go through again.

I was in Conifer Park. I had been there for ten days when my counselor came around and told me, "Sylvia," he said, "we feel that you should go to a half-way house." And I'm like, "Whoah." "Well, we think that you'd have a better chance." I'm like, "I'm not going to no half-way house. I've been here ten days and I don't need no half-way house. I'll be cured when I go home, blah, blah, blah." I was so upset that they suggested something like that. I jumped on the phone and I called my mother. Then I called my brother and thank God I have a level-headed brother. He turned around and said, "Sylvia, stop and think about it. If you don't go into a half-way house, to at least get a little bit more knowledge about what it is that's bothering you," he said, "what's going to happen even six months from now?" And I said, "Well, all right. I'll give it a try." I went back to my counselor and I told my counselor okay. I said, "I talked it over with my mother and I talked it over with my brother and I've come to a decision. I'm going to a half-way house under one condition: that I don't have to move to a half-way house in New York." So he said, "No problem."

I came here to Springfield, Massachusetts, to Temple Street, to Ethos House. I came here May 8th of 1987. Eight months later, I graduated from Ethos and moved into my first apartment I ever had sober. I used to talk to my mother at least two or three times a week and I'll never forget what we were talking about. I had started working for Childworld in July of '87, where I still work at now. This particular Christmas of '87 they had just came out with what they call the Muppet Puppets. They had Miss Piggy and Kermit, and I had bought my own Miss Piggy. I was telling my mother about it and my mother said she wanted one. And she said, "If they come in, get me one and I'll send you the money." I told her she could have mine. Both my brothers were coming up to spend my first Christmas in my new apartment with me, here in Massachusetts.

One morning, cable was supposed to come at nine o'clock. Of course, cable didn't come, and so I was on the phone with my friend Marty. As I say, the Lord works in mysterious ways. If cable had gotten there at nine o'clock like they were supposed to, I might not have been home to get the phone call. I was on the phone with my girlfriend, and I have call waiting, and the phone beeped. I said, "Well, hold on, Marty, I've got another call coming in." It was my oldest brother and he says, "Sylvia, I got something to tell you." I could tell from his voice that something was wrong. It didn't dawn on me: my mother. My mother was dead. I was thinking my father, but he told me my mother died. I went into hysterics.

To this day I do not know what caused me to pick up the phone to call my sponsor. I also called this fellow Pete who had been in the house with me and had graduated a couple of months before me. He had given me his job number and his home number. I called him at his job. He asked me did I want to go to New York that night. I told him, "I want to go but I can't go until the morning when I can go to the bank and take the money out of the bank." He told me, "Don't worry about your money." Pete gave me money, made sure if I needed anything that I'd be able to take care of it. He drove me at four o'clock that afternoon. Two o'clock we got the call, two hours later, we're on the road heading to New York.

Do you ever feel cheated? Do you ever feel, "Why me?"

Yes. Maybe I shouldn't try to analyze everything, but I guess a part of me, I try to see, why do I feel cheated? Maybe it's something

I did. I stop and think about it. Even now, as of March 3rd, 1991, Lord willing, I'll be clean and sober for four years. I don't care what A.A. preaches, or N.A., or whoever it is, there's always going to be a time that no matter how good you're doing, no matter how much you get into it, that you're still going to have problems when things don't go your way. Why me? Because even now when I'm sober for years I don't have the excuse where if I hadn't of drank those two shots of bourbon last night or if I hadn't of smoked that last joint last night, I wouldn't feel like this. Now I have to sit down and try to figure out, why am I still feeling like this? There's times in my life when I feel like I've had a drink, when I actually feel like I've got a hangover and don't know why.

I'm learning, slowly but surely. I'm just getting into a step meeting. It took me a long, long time to accept that I am a recovering alcoholic and a recovering drug addict. I have a sickness, I have a disease that will not go away. It's like if you get cancer, there's no guarantee that you're going to beat cancer. So I have to deal with it day by day. I have to accept day by day that I cannot drink, I cannot pick up a drug. I go to meetings for the simple reason I know throughout my whole being that if I pick up a drug I will die. I got to go to A.A. because if I ever relapse, if I get lost and think, "Well, one drink won't hurt me. . . . "

September 1990

Laura

Thirty-nine years old, she lives in a small town outside of Boston, Massachusetts. The apartment she shares with Lisa, her lover, consists of five rooms in a renovated historical house. Books of poetry, books about women and by women overflow onto end tables and chairs. She is five feet seven, and has short cropped hair. At times she looks tense, her emotions seem raw, fragmented. Sexually abused by her father, emotionally abused by her mother, Laura perseveres. "We were poor. For me, Pancake House was not a treat. That was dinner." Both of her parents are alcoholics. She has been writing poetry since she was seven. She works as a paste-up artist. She attends Alcoholics Anonymous and Al-Anon. She has been sober since 1981.

I'm an incest survivor. I know from therapy—and it's just been confirmed by my mother—that the incest started when I was eighteen months old. My mom went downstairs to get coffee or to get the paper and came back to find my father trying to shove his penis in my mouth. I was eighteen months old. I was sitting on the bed. My Mom was eight months pregnant with a baby she ended up losing.

There was so much arguing in the house and I felt responsible for it. I would hear my parents fighting. It was violent. I started having fainting spells when I was in second grade. My dad wore a uniform where he worked and I would faint at the sight of security guards, crossing guards, and policemen. I was given medication very early, so I learned to pop pills at an early age.

On Christmas Day, when I was seven, my mother, my sister and

I left my father. There had been a bad incident on Christmas Eve with my father really snapping out. No one would talk about what was going on. That rule of nobody talking got so enforced. You drank problems away and you ate them away, and you pilled them away. You'd pop something in your mouth to make yourself feel better and you wouldn't verbalize anything. Nobody ever explained what the hell was going on.

My dad was gone and it was the first divorce or separation in our little Catholic neighborhood. By the time I got to high school, divorce was happening more often, but we were the first and it got me special privileges. We were like stray cats but I was able to milk that for all it was worth.

My mom went to work. This was in the fifties and she got $25 a week alimony for the two of us. I mean, that's really fuckin' shit. I've seen her paycheck too; she was working for Travelers [an insurance company], which is notoriously one of the worst-paying companies for women.

"That Ruth woman with her trampy little daughters." It's like nobody was wrapped too tight, sexually or otherwise, in my household. We had the pedophilc sick father and then the lesbian mother who starts going out with my lover. We have my poor sister who maybe really is straight but trying to make sense of all this. And I was a hippy dippy.

I remember drinking Cold Duck when I was thirteen and getting very drunk, thinking I was really cool. I still want it. It's been eight years and I still want a beer. My mother said it was my craving for beer when she was pregnant with me that got her hooked on it. She wanted me to learn to drink at home so I would be prepared to drink out in the world. I think one of the roles I played in her life was to be a drinking buddy.

I went to a Catholic high school. I got a better education but I learned to be sneakier. My coming out incident happened when I was thirteen. My best friend, who was a freshman, invited me to her birthday party. I was the only person invited to sleep over and she made love to me. I guess I was one of the birthday presents. I liked it, but that became another secret, another thing I didn't talk about.

I had been programmed to go to college somewhere along the line. I went to a Catholic women's college. One night I told my best friend, my roommate, that I was in love with her. I got kicked out of college for being a lesbian.

I had a few sexual encounters with men. When I saw the penis, particularly if they wanted me to give them oral sex, I would throw up. Violently throw up. I always blamed that on the booze. I never realized that something else had been going on with that until I got sober. That was my father's thing. I can remember my mother, when I was thirteen or fourteen, telling me how my father would want her to do that for him and she wouldn't do it. That was one of his problems. It was inappropriate for my mom to tell a kid that. I already knew it was one of his problems because I was probably the one who was doing it for him. I *still* block that out.

I haven't seen my father since I was twenty-two and my sister was nineteen. She needed four hundred dollars for a brake job. She asked him for it and he said he would lend her the money if she would blow him. I can remember her coming home hysterical. I wrote him off then. He went on sending birthday presents and money at Christmas. I sent the money back and said I wanted nothing to do with him.

My mother came out with one of my lovers—more of the soap opera. I really don't think she was physical with me. It was more like emotional incest. The fact that she slept with lovers of mine—I remember her saying that she hadn't been with anyone for seventeen years, male or female, and that was the sacrifice she made for me and my sister. I remember thinking, "That is so sick." Seventeen years without sex or companionship, and our house had always been like a haven for battered and deserted women in the neighborhood.

I found a lesbian bar. Actually, my mom found it. I thought I had died and gone to heaven. I remember needing to get very drunk to go there. My mom had picked out somebody for me at the bar that was going to be the perfect person, and she was, because she was the bartender. Her name was Sandy. It's what any alcoholic would fall in love with. Sandy thought my mother and I were lovers when we walked in there together. She thought we were trying to set her up for some kind of strange scene. It was very bizarre. We fell in love, or something like it, and she moved into my mother's house.

By this time, my sister had gone bananas a couple of times. She didn't have an alcohol problem; she had a Valium addiction. She was militantly straight. I can appreciate where she's coming from with the three other family members being quote unquote perverted.

I started to hang out at the bar a lot. This was the height of disco, and the place became the hottest women-owned disco in town. Sandy became manager and everything was perfect. My life became that bar. It really revolved around partying and working second shift. I got into speed and uppers a lot and my whole life was, get out of work at midnight, and go down to the bar. Since she was the manager, the serious stuff didn't start until after everyone had left at one or two in the morning. I would be there 'til five or six, go home, and pass out for a while. I can remember that she had a big gavel. We always had to make sure the gavel was filled for the first hit in the morning before we got out of bed. The speed and the beer were already lined up. It was just really insane.

My mom was still doing her thing. We had an open relationship because that was politically correct. But we didn't have to try to be politically correct. We were just bar dykes.

Easter of 1976, I had my first registered psychotic break. I remember I was starting to get a little bit involved with the Women's Center, which is a more political crowd. I was reading a gay American history book. My mom was seeing a woman who lived in New Haven and worked for the state, so they were very hush, hush, undercover with their stuff and didn't really like to come to the bars that much. It was Easter weekend and I remember going down to the bar. I had called an ex-lover who had confronted me about my drinking. She had moved to San Francisco and I didn't know it. Nobody else was around that night and I went down to the bar and I remember I just wanted to talk to my mom. Having this open relationship, Sandy told me she wasn't coming home that night. I met another girlfriend but she was busy, too. I remember having three Jack Daniels that night. Everybody was saying, "What's the matter? Have a Jack Daniels, you'll feel better."

I went home and started reading a gay American history book in our nice suburban little house and suddenly I began trashing my mother's house all night long. I was hallucinating really badly. Partly from reading the gay history book, I thought the house was surrounded and that there were people shooting. I was running from window to window.

You remember all that?

Yeah, kind of. I kind of remember how it felt. I was having this psychotic break. I got in my car at six o'clock on Easter morning.

I had a nice bottle of wine and I was going up to my mother's in New Hampshire to have Easter dinner. I just kept driving and ran out of gas right over the Massachusetts line. I was still hallucinating but I remember the cops. They just wanted to see if I was okay. I was bananas. I insisted they get a matron.

So here it is, Easter Sunday. I'm in this little tiny town refusing to get in the cops' car. I have my lover's license on me instead of mine and she's at her parents' house for Easter dinner. She gets a phone call from the cops in New Hampshire saying she's in New Hampshire. And here's her crazy-assed lover somewhere in the next state with her license.

They were going through my wallet trying to find out who I was and who they could get in touch with. Finally, they talked to Sandy and she called a couple of people at the bar trying to find out where my mom might be. Of course nobody knew. So then we had a big rescue thing. Sandy came to get me. It was already nighttime by then and she drove my car back and friends come to take me home. I ended up getting put in a nuthouse.

I was committed in Boston. That started in '76 and went on for five years. Every time I was committed they called it a "psychotic break." I was never called an alcoholic. I was called "schizophrenic," "psychotic," "psychotic-depressive," and every other label. I was on psychotropic drugs—Stelazine, Thorazine, whatever. I know it's a miracle that I survived, because I continued to drink. Every time they put me in the hospital, which was only a few blocks away from the bar, I would get a two-hour pass and I'd head for the bar. That was home to me and that's what the next five years were about.

Do you think the alcohol triggered the psychotic breaks?

Yeah, definitely. The last hospitalization I had I woke up in a black-out. I was strapped down. I don't know how I got there. Nobody else seems to know how I got there or what happened. But I was committed and it took my mom and a lawyer a month to get me uncommitted and transferred to a regular hospital. By that time, I had pneumonia. I mean, that was backward time. It was a snake pit.

What's that like?

Where they lock the doors. It was a locked ward where people walked around screaming. It was bedlam, you know. It was like the worst nightmare.

That doesn't exist anymore, does it?

No, thank God. Now it's a detox. I went down to speak at an A.A. meeting in recovery and it was really scary, one of the scariest things I ever did, because of my memories of how it was. They said I looked totally freaked out when I stood up at the podium. I really thought I was going to lose it. But I needed to get over the fear of a place that doesn't exist anymore. I never even belonged there.

All through this I was writing poetry, which I've been doing from the time I was in second grade. I was always creative, both verbally and in my writing. My first hospitalization, that Easter hospitalization, was the year Sylvia Plath's movie, *The Bell Jar*, was made. *The Boston Phoenix* had a contest for women poets in conjunction with that opening and I won second place. I ended up in a mental hospital instead, so I couldn't go to get the prize, which was an autographed copy of Sylvia's book *The Bell Jar*, which I wish I had. It was a big contest.

My poem didn't get published. The first prize was getting published in *The Boston Phoenix*, which was the big alternative paper back then. I remember having a shrink who was just amazed with my creativity. All of this was part of the Sylvia Plath/Anne Sexton syndrome. I was thought to have the same kind of ability. The last poem I ever had published was published anonymously in a psychiatric journal as evidence of creativity in a schizophrenic. It was something that I wrote in therapy while in the hospital. We were all shuffling around. I remember they had it hanging on the bulletin board of the psych ward, right by the cafeteria. It was posted without my name on it.

During my last hospitalization, they took me off of every medication. I was in a padded room. I was in a padded room and I had six shock treatments, but I wasn't on any medication.

What does it feel like to have shock treatment?

I don't know because they always gave you a shot before. The thing I hated the most was, because that's a teaching hospital, there would be twenty people in the room watching me. I'm grateful, I never experienced memory loss from it, but I also didn't gain anything—I don't know, maybe I did gain something. I still didn't talk, it didn't make me open up. I reverted to an infant. I had a primary nurse who was feeding me Enfamil, a protein drink, because I thought food was poison. My mom would bring me McDonald's cheeseburgers and I'd toss them. I thought they were poisoned. I was still pretty delusionary. I had to be spoon-fed and held, but I came back. Something happened and I really don't know what. I wasn't on drugs, I wasn't on anything. When I got released from the hospital, it was Memorial Day 1981.

And that's your sobriety anniversary?

No, it's not really. It's my sanity. It took me a little longer to get into recovery. When I got released from the hospital, I started to see a therapist every day, because by that time I had been institutionalized so much that I was not very functional. They said I would need intensive follow-up. I didn't want to work with the shrink who thought I was reincarnated or something. I knew stuff was getting weird. A therapist named Jan agreed to work with me. I was on welfare and living at my mom's house. I didn't have a lover but I was still hanging around at the bar. I was drinking beer but I wasn't using drugs. Jan had made a contract with me as a therapist that I would not use street drugs of any sort too, as well as not being on a 'script. So this was the first time since I had been put on phenobarbital that I wasn't using a prescribed substance.

I went to the Voluntary Action Council Center and signed up for a job. It turned out to be on the Commission on the Status of Women that had been started by the governor. It was a small state agency. I helped with collating. When I started, there were five women who worked in the office. I started to regain something. I saw the therapist, went over to the volunteer job, and I started to get something back. I had one more break while I was there. I ended up with a real short hospitalization, and again, I don't really know what happened.

When I got out, they had managed to get a grant for me to be a paid employee of the state. I was amazed. I'm still amazed. I had regained some of the skills that I had lost.

It was the early eighties and politicians were playing nice. In September there was a conference and they picked me to represent the Commission on the Status of Women, at this lesbian and gay conference. I went to it and one of the coordinators of the conference had a really distinctive voice. I went up to her afterwards and found that I knew her from the bars and that she had been going to a program called Overeaters Anonymous.

By that time, I weighed about 220 pounds. I was immense. I would cop to maybe food was an issue. The therapist had said not to use street drugs. I think I did one more acid trip. My therapist was in Al-Anon and ACOA. She kept trying to steer me into Al-Anon because of my mom's drinking. We focused on that a lot in therapy. There was a big hole that I could see myself in, or that I was going to fall into. I would faint sometimes in her office. I never talked about the incest with her. I never worked any of that through then. I went to Overeaters Anonymous.

On Labor Day weekend I went to a women's music retreat. I took a sleeping bag and a case of beer in a cooler. When I got up there, the woman who is now my sponsor was walking around with a button that said, *"I Like Sober Dykes."* I'm thinking, "What is going on here?" There was a sign on one of the trees near the crafts area that said "Friends of Bill W. meeting here," and I'm going, why do they have a man's name at a women's conference? I'm like, what does this mean?

I'm sitting there listening to this woman do her songs and some of them talked about the old days from the bar, and she also had this new stuff about being free and having choices. I thought, what? I had already come into O.A. and I remember going home that night and cracking open a beer and saying, "I wonder if I might have a problem with anything other than food?"

This was the first time you knew?

Yes, but I cracked open a beer to think about it. Her story was too similar. She was secretly gay from high school. She also mentioned alcohol being a problem, that she'd been two and half years without a drink or a drug. I was getting closer and closer to putting it down, but I just didn't want to cop to it. I was much safer feeling like food was the issue. I was crazy Laura, I'm psychotic. And everyone knew me as being a real jerk-off mental case. I preferred that. *Please* don't tell me that I'm not going to be able to drink or drug. I had already copped to not drugging. Now they're going to take the last good thing away? Unh-uh.

But my thirtieth birthday was coming up and my self-esteem was really coming back from having that job, too, you know—being involved in women's issues for the state. We were putting conferences together and I was really utilizing some skills and getting brain cells back. Grandiose alcoholic that I was, and still sometimes can be, I wanted to have thirty women for my thirtieth birthday party. I was told to invite forty to ensure that I had the thirty. So I did. My birthday is November 15 and I talked a friend into going to an A.A. meeting.

She had the bigger problem of course, and it took her a month before she went to A.A., to the lesbian meeting with me. I stopped drinking the day before we went to that meeting. She stopped that day. Her sobriety date is November 11 and mine is November 10.

I didn't remember my birthdays from forever. I know I had them. I was just too messed up to remember them. I had invited forty women and there were thirty-eight women and one man because the director of the Commission on the Status of Women was going out with a man and she actually brought her boyfriend. He was cool, you know. It was a bizarre party.

I was five days sober. There were friends I had made from the program, people were doing drugs in my bedroom, people were drinking, there were friends from the bar who brought me champagne, and I got a case of Heineken. But I didn't drink. Somebody brought me an ounce of coke and I just handed the shit back. I was cleaning someone's puke up at four in the morning. The party was at my mother's house and she was shit-faced. Some of her older dyke friends had come to the kid's party. That was kind of how I was treated. But it was this real blast. I still have alcoholic or drunken dyke friends who say, "God, when are you going to have another party like your thirtieth?"

They're still drinking?

Yeah, and I'll run into that. I had been trying to track Sandy down, to have her come to the party. A week after my birthday, she called. She was drunk and she was going to drive her father's car off this cliff. I talked her down. She was drunk and she was standing up there in a phone booth calling to say goodbye. She had a fifth of vodka. I said, "Your father will fucking kill you if you drive his Oldsmobile off the cliff. He will kill you. You'd better die." She started laughing and that did it. She was fine.

What do you think is so seductive about that—suicide, drama?

There's a whole scenario of that being seductively cool. Even when you're drunk, it just seems so romantic or something. I don't know. It's the whole creativity thing. The Sylvia Plath/Anne Sexton thing. I tried to kill my mother once.

Seriously, with a knife or a gun or something?

Knife. I would get homicidal. That was the thing, I would get psychotic. I kicked Sandy's windshield in in front of the bar 'cause she was leaving with somebody else. Just the tragedy of it all.

Do you ever feel like it's the same path, going down a real codependent path?

Oh yeah. If I don't take care of my codependency now, that's what I'm going to drink over. That's what will lead me back to drinking and that's why I work the other programs that I do. Because I think that codependency is the issue. And, for me, the incest too. It's like if I don't heal beyond that, I'm going to drink again.

I met Lisa at an A.A. meeting. It was my third year. She needed help. My little codependent, caretaking heart just went nuts. I remember going up to her after the meeting. She came down a couple

of weeks later to the Wednesday night lesbian meeting. At the break
I asked her if she wanted a hug. August 1 was our lovers' anniversary,
but I met her in March and I kept telling her. . . . She wanted to go
to bed with me and I kept saying, "You need a friend right now."
She was trying to get out of a relationship. Nobody had ever said
that to her. There was something about her: I didn't want it to be a
one-night stand. I didn't want it to be the rescue fuck. That's what
I kept arguing with her about. We've gone through a lot in the last
six years. She has been with other people. I haven't, and when people
find out they say, "Wow, this program works."

Have you ever forgiven your father?

I don't feel like I have to. I don't have to forgive anything. That's
not anywhere near . . . I mean, I have a real hard time with Adult
Children of Alcoholics. When you go to ACOA, "They did the best
they could with what they got." Yeah, bullshit. They did really
fucked up things and I'm not beyond that myself at eight years sober.
No way.

What would you recommend an incest survivor do, a woman?

Al-Anon, ACOA is another. There are some incest survivors
meetings which are real intense, and there's individual therapy. Al-
Anon is definitely getting more open to talking about those issues.
I've heard both men and women talk about those issues. I go to
straight Al-Anon meetings and I'm really amazed that they've opened
up to so much.

Do you think codependency is harder than the alcohol?

Yes, because it's the people, the people addiction and it's come
pretty close. The closest I've ever come to wanting to die and the
closest I've ever come to wanting to drink is around the relationship,
when things were not good between us. Over the last six years,
things have gotten pretty bad.

I've been going to one particular Al-Anon meeting for two years. I would hear people saying in that room that when you're constantly caretaking, you're not letting people have the dignity to live their life. I couldn't fathom what they were talking about. It's like, "They are helpless fools, they need me, don't you understand?" It's not true. Lisa knows how to do lots of stuff. A gay man from my Monday night meeting, who has been sober forever, said, "Who asked you? Who asked you to do this stuff? She's not asking you to do this stuff, to take it all on. You're snapping out under the pressure. Did you ever ask her?" No, I didn't. I was just like doing this stuff thinking that I was supposed to be doing it. That's codependency and that's the killing thing. I think I am getting a grip on that from Al-Anon and from therapy and from working my A.A. program and the steps.

I remember going to Al-Anon and saying, "I don't care if every one of you in this room loves me tonight, she doesn't love me tonight, so the hell with you. I don't care." And now, I hear myself saying, "I'm here tonight because I know everyone in this room loves me and if she doesn't love me tonight, that's her problem and it's really too bad. That's her loss." Plus I've had sponsors tell me I can't go crazy any more, I've already done that. I use food, you know, Ben and Jerry's. I've had a lot of one night stands with Ben and Jerry and just eaten myself into a stupor.

The biggest lesson I've learned in the past eight and a half years is that this is all a process. I'm always amazed when speakers in A.A. say, "A.A. gave me back my life." Well, I never *got* a life. I had no role models and I had no guidelines. Now I have the steps and I have people I can ask for help. I can talk on the phone and I can do the stuff I'm supposed to do. I can help other people and not have control over them.

I can't imagine not going to A.A. I don't want to not go to A.A., but I don't consider that a measure of wellness, necessarily. Although I want to get on with my life and do healthy, lively things without checking where it came from.

There are a lot of women who are dually addicted and a lot of women who've been misdiagnosed, who are chronic psych patients. You don't have to be. I'm grateful that I self-diagnosed. I've had people in recovery who just don't believe that they don't have to be mental. They don't connect with it because they're so used to that label. I definitely enjoyed that label a lot more, too. I thought insanity was a good excuse to do what I did.

I had this shrink, I ran into him when I was six months sober and he asked me what I was doing. It was at a concert and I told to him, that I was six months sober in A.A. and he said to me, yet again, "Oh, um, well, I think once you work out your psychological problems you can probably safely drink again." I went to my Monday night A.A. meeting and I told them that and people in the room said, "You decide to pick up again, you call him and take him with you. Take him on a night of drinking with you and he will see."

Lisa knows me so well. She'll look at me and say, "You've got your incest face on," or "Where are you?"

There was a guy that used to say, "A.A. doesn't promise you a new car, a new job, and a new girlfriend." I used to sit there and say, "I got a new car, a new job, and a new girlfriend." I didn't know what the hell he was talking about. I've also lost some of those things in A.A., but I still have my sobriety. If we just stay clean and sober, anything is possible—beyond our wildest dreams. I have enough respect for where alcohol has taken me, it terrifies me. There are thirty other people in my life now. If I can spread it out among thirty people in my A.A. group, *nobody* is going to get burned out.

August 1990

Part Four

In Love

If being in love is to be suddenly united with
the most unruly, the most outrageously alive
part of yourself, this state of piercing
consciousness did not subside in me, as I've
learned it does in others. . . . If my mind could
have made a sound, it would have burst a
row of wineglasses. I saw coincidences
everywhere. . . . This agony, this delight did
not recede. . . .

—Scott Spencer,
Endless Love

Margaret

She is twenty-five years old. Her father is a well-known graphic artist. Her sister graduated from Yale. "I was the pretty one, and she was the smart one." Margaret used drugs and alcohol to dull her intensity but now she feels robbed and works on her recovery at a gut level, paying herself back. A vulnerable woman, she lives in Brooklyn and appears outwardly tough to shield herself from some of the violence and despair she sees every day in New York City. While she is complicated and analytical, a part of her longs to be simple. "People never said, 'You're a young girl, why don't you enjoy being young?' Everyone said, 'Wow, you're an intense, intuitive young gorgeous girl and we like having you around.' " Her father is an alcoholic. She works as a waitress in Manhattan. She has been sober since October of 1989. This interview has been broken into two parts, as Margaret had only been sober for a few months when I first met her, and wanted to be interviewed again, after she had been sober for a year.

Well, the bottom line is I lived in Manhattan until I was six. It was the raw part of Manhattan, like when people who did dope were crouching on corners. I lived on the Upper East Side and I went to your typical public East Side grade school.

My mother's from Austria and moved here when Hitler hit the fan. She was lucky and she knows it. She came from a Jewish background and met my dad at an advertising agency. My father was a powerful guy and thought that he was really intense. He was probably totally insecure on the inside.

My mother lived for her kids and her husband, and he wanted a dream. His dream was to deny the fact that he enjoyed making a lot of money. So he moved us to the country. He just picked us all up and moved us to this little dumb-fuck town upstate with nothing: a school with three hundred kids from first through twelfth grade. We lived on a resort in the boonies. The town opened up in the summer and shut down in the winter, but had eight bars in it along one little strip with one stoplight. Basically everyone knew what you had for dinner the day before you had it and that was just something you had to deal with. It was totally uncultured, ridiculous. The school library and the town library consisted of Nancy Drew. That's what they believed was life. Unfortunately I hung out with people who believed that and will make it in life believing that. But they'll miss out.

I didn't grow up with a religion. We had a Christmas tree on Christmas and a menorah on Jewish holidays. I'm glad because I don't fight a Higher Power. I'm more than happy to let it be a mystery. I don't need to have it written down, I don't need to be manipulated. I know I didn't get here because I'm God and some God hurt me. I like the way Indians talk: they call it the Great Mystery.

When I was younger my older sister and I were extremely close. I looked up to her totally. She did really cool things. She really loved her books. She tried to help me but I rebelled against her.

I was born with a pretty face, and it was a hindrance. I lost my virginity when I was eleven and a half. I remember making out with guys when I was younger, thinking, I want more. I wanted an orgasm. These young guys in sixth grade didn't know how to tongue-kiss right. I thought, "There's got to be more to this shit." I met a guy who was from Colorado and we started making love. All we ever did was screw. I had my first orgasm when I was twelve, and I loved it. I was into masturbating. I think I just felt comfortable that way.

When I was nine I picked up my first drink. I was never drunk when I had sex, it wasn't like that. I knew exactly what was going on. I used to try to deny it and say, "It was when I was drunk." But no, sex was a real feeling. I started getting traces of wanting alcohol when I was about nine.

My dad would get really drunk, and when my parents got divorced my mother met somebody whom she could love and who would be there for her. My mother got a divorce because she realized that my father was doing what *he* wanted to do, and that was wrong. You have to care about your partner in life. My mother taught me that. My father really hurt my mother. She had done what she thought was the right thing, which was to go with him and to try to make a life in this little dumb town, and my mother is a really brilliant, caring woman.

In school I was different. There was a little crowd that I ended up finding. After four months the guy that I was dating dumped me because I wasn't willing to get high. I was just scared. He broke my heart, and in the meantime told someone in that tiny little town that we had sex. So I went down as the school slut. There were a couple of us school sluts and we didn't go near each other but we knew who we were. The sad thing is we weren't sluts. We just wanted to experience life.

I always felt things at a really young age. I understood other people's feelings and it was hard for me to buy into society. My father started drinking even more when my mother left. We went bankrupt and we had to move back to New York. My father knew how to make money as an art director and a graphic artist. When we got to the city, I realized I couldn't live with him because he would say such mean things to me. He rejected me because I looked like my mother. I think he was just in so much pain. I was an easy target, and was very hurt. My sister and I moved in with my mother. My sister went to college, to Yale, and I lived in the room that we used to share and had it as my own.

My father kind of drifted off. I basically just didn't bother with him for a long time, which was probably better for me anyway. When I was growing up he always told me things—that guys were going to feel up my shirt, and call me a slut—and in a sense his gruesome thoughts came true. The thing is, he didn't say it like he wanted to watch out for me, he said it for shock value. People have weird reasons for telling you things when you're young. I think sometimes they enjoy hearing themselves sounding like they know shit, but their motives are just greasy. I don't know how else to explain it.

So I'm in the city, in junior high, and I end up meeting kids that smoke pot and get high and listen to the kind of music I listen to. My stepfather was about twenty years younger than my mother in a sixties kind of way. He never got high, but he was into really good music. I ended up being a young little hippie girl. I ran around and cut school and became a vegetarian and got high. They put me in a dumb class because I was from upstate. I had to prove to them that I was smart. I was doing all right in school. I went to Music and Art.

I ended up getting along better with some of the teachers than I did the students. I couldn't take being around kids my own age. I was really into my own life even though it was weird. Now I realize it was just my life.

I chose to get drunk and high on a constant basis. I met kids my own age but a lot of them thought I was kind of weird. I was pretty, so men were constantly on my ass to be with them. And of course, I fell in love with them. That became an easy thing to do. I'm a warm, loving, caring person and it's easy to get taken advantage of.

I ended up moving in and out of home several times. I ended up living at my mother's house for three years with a guy who was a total hippie and introduced me to acid. The drinking had kind of subsided. I was into health food and drugs.

I saw my father only three times a year, for holidays. My mother and my stepfather were really good to me. As much as I chose to run around and be really wild, they were kind and loving and supportive and I have to remember that all the time.

My sister freaked out that I was involved in this weird drug underworld. I dove right into it. I did things that white kids from good homes did in the early seventies . . . like go and write graffiti everywhere, and go to parties and get high, and talk about philosophy; it was like a strange subculture.

I ended up living with a guy who was a kung fu specialist. He taught me about Buddhism and things that now I can carry with me in life, like yin and yang, things I already knew, but he enhanced them. It turned out that he was a jerk. People love to claim to be spiritual.

I moved in and out so many different times, staying with various people. I always ended up back at home, with my tail between my legs. Yet I was sort of abusive. My mother would lend me money, or give me money, and I would spend it all on getting high or drunk.

Then I met a girlfriend and we dove into the weird club scene here, because we were both young and pretty. We were writing graffiti and we thought we were cool and we hung out with all these Latin kids. We were tough and I started drug dealing on the side.

Basically I began to make a bottom for myself. I was walking down the ladder.

Did you know it?

Yeah, in the back of my mind. Yet I always thought that I wouldn't be one of those people that gets addicted to alcohol or drugs. But I did. My life was fucking crazy. It was painful. Even the cool hippie types and the weird Latin types I met, they just didn't understand me. I was in a weird class all by myself. Today I'm glad about that. These people who just want to be in molds, they're just so fucking *lame*.

I really ran. I really had a crazy, crazy time. I was out there. I was getting drunk. I was going to clubs, and I would get in free. I was an *in, young, graffiti-type chick,* on the *scene*. I stayed out a couple of nights a week and on weekends. I would meet people and, you know, just be a nut job. I was happy with it.

I moved into my girlfriend's apartment with her father and her crazy Methadone-addict brother. We were really crazy and yet we were always safe. We led a really safe existence.

My sister found out at one point and became really scared for me. It's hard to have people tell you that they want to help you. At that age I was so rebellious and she didn't understand. I continued to get high and drink. Smoking pot was near and dear to me, I really enjoyed it. I smoked so much pot, took hallucinogens and crazy stuff. I was still out partying all the time and then my girlfriend ended up getting involved with a guy who I really didn't like. I kind of stepped away from that. I was getting high a lot more and I didn't really want to bother with people.

I met this guy Eric and we moved in together. Actually we fucked for about two years, living at my mother's. I felt that I truly liked him and he loved me, because I was such a rebel. He came from a good Spanish home, supposedly. I felt that I wanted to change for him. I thought that if I grew my nails, and brushed my hair, and ate meat, and did normal things that I wouldn't be such a nut job.

I envisioned so much. My gut instincts were always so right about people, and that scared me. I always felt weird and different and overly spiritual. I remember saying to my girlfriend, "You know I just want somebody simple to get involved with. *Please,* just let me be simple."

Little did I know that this simple thing would become a complex burden. The first few years were good and then it just went downhill. I denied who I was. I like eating well, I like talking about spiritual stuff, I like talking about mysticism, and how God is a mystery. I'm grateful that I'm sober, but I'm not grateful for how I got here. I understand and respect and accept why, but I just don't believe that almighty, saintly shit.

During all of that I had three abortions, none of which I feel bad about. I feel bad in a sense that it shouldn't have happened but I wouldn't change it. If you're pretty, everybody thinks life should be good. You must have guys clamoring around you to pay your way and do all this shit. But why would you want anyone to pay your way . . . I mean, what the fuck is that? Nobody believes a pretty girl feels down.

I really just wanted someone to accept who I was and listen to me. I was always searching for the right guy to give me an honest answer to whatever question . . . I don't even know what the fuck the question was, or the answer. But I was always searching. Everything was right there in front of me. I was a very special chosen woman. I just chose not to believe that and let myself feel insecure.

The drugging and the drinking became progressively—in such a bad space, the only thing left for me to do was to really get introverted, which I wholeheartedly did. I never came out and said I was in pain. I never told anybody anything.

I remember just before I got clean, I would cry to my boyfriend to accept me and try to change his ways. But he was a control freak. He would get drunk and get fucked up and then feel bad about it. I think the bottom line about my childhood was that it just wasn't typical. I don't know if people stopped me from enjoying my childhood, or if I stopped me, or if I chose to be an adult at an early age or whatever the fuck it was, but that's what happened. I wanted to run hard and run strong. I would read books on Janis Joplin and all these sixties people and think, God, they know what I'm feeling. They know that it's hard to be different. Today I'm learning about even sicker and more intense people. There are people out there that hurt.

I ended up in places that I should not have been at a young age. I'm not searching for my childhood anymore because I'll never have that back. But at least I can gently caress the child that's still in me, that needs every now and then to jump up and down, and shriek, or feel really bad or guilty, or feel nothing.

March 1990

The reason I drank and drugged was because I wanted to find God. I was on a bizarre path, like some stupid Carlos Castañeda junkie. I thought that the more I took drugs and drank, the closer I would get to some experience with a Higher Power. And A.A. has given me a God of my understanding. I am a Christian, but I don't care what the hell anyone else is.

You're not going to be lighting the Chanukah candles on Tuesday?

Fuck, no. Most organized religions suck. I don't go to churches, I don't. I take the Bible as the word of God.

What is your definition of spirituality?

Spirituality is respecting that you are not the power greater than anything—It's making a really good attempt to practice all your principles. Outside of the program it's taking time for myself, sitting with myself quietly and not being afraid of the noise in my head. Which I can't say that I always do, but I try. It's being good to people, even if I don't really like them. I respect where they are coming from. It's listening to the small things; leaves in the wind, my dog sleeping, which is nice stuff. Stuff that counts. Respecting every tiny little thing. Knowing that I can't be perfect, but I can try.

I pray for guidance and the will to do the right thing, not self-will run rampant. The city is like a penitentiary—it's really hard. Recently, with the grace of God, working, and my parents' help, I was able to get a garden apartment with a fireplace. It reminds me of upstate New York where I used to live and that's nice.

Can you think of any circumstance under which you would start drinking again?

No. No, I can't. A.A. has really made it hard for me. I can go off on a run mentally where I'm a big asshole. I don't do anything right. I'm willful and try to think of nasty things to do, dark things that aren't good for me. Basically A.A. has taught me that whatever has gone down, I can use the steps, or something I've heard, or a slogan: *Easy Does It, Let Go and Let God,* things that I used to loathe. Even now, *Easy Does It* and I don't get along too well, but I pray to understand that slogan more. There are other times when I want to be such a bitch and be awful and just really go crazy sexually or mentally, or physically hurt somebody. The city starts to get to me. And then I think about what I've learned. Then it's like A.A. has really done a number on anything fucked-up I want to do.

I guess being spiritual isn't pretending to be better than you are. Sometimes I just have to feel whatever I am feeling. I have trouble with that, I always think I am supposed to label it, analyze it and *know* it. The thing that's been happening in my sobriety is that I am really working . . . I go to therapy outside of A.A. because I need to discuss personal issues that I don't think I should discuss in the rooms.*

I really need professional help and my therapist now is helping me retrace my childhood and talk about the first feelings I had. The first feeling I ever had was fear. I think fear is really a big inhibitor. I think it really gets alcoholics going. The fear of change, even if it's good change, I'm scared of it. A girlfriend of mine, since she did her fourth and fifth steps, she doesn't care what she talks about in the rooms. She will talk about anything. I have to tip my hat to her. I really do, but that's not me.

You've done your fourth and fifth [A.A. steps], haven't you?

I did it in a weird way. I did steps one through seven in one night at an A.A. fix-it. That was heavy. I had trouble doing my third step on my knees and screaming. I don't think God needs me to scream. It was real good for me because it taught me a lot about the original

*The rooms imply A.A. meetings.

A.A. But I'm doing another fourth step that's in more detail. My first fourth step was a just a laundry list. I want to get more into why and how and when.

I hope one day I can move up to a mountain and, like they say in Alaska, there are eight men to every women. What more could you ask for? I'll have a whole harem.

Do you think you were as addicted to men as you were to alcohol?

No, I'm not as addicted to men as I thought I was. I get one man and I'm addicted to him for a long period of time. In sobriety I've only had sex with three people. For someone who has had major sex, I thought I would have been dogging my ass off. But it's different now. I can't condone that sort of thing in me. I have a lot of sex issues that I have to deal with. My therapist thinks I was sexually abused verbally as a child. Not physically, but verbally, like knowing too much. Well, I heard Bradshaw say it on TV. I thought, "Oh great, Bradshaw is on TV again." *The inner child, the inner child. . . .* And I agree, everything does go back to the child in you. But sometimes I just want to tell everybody to fuck off.

I was talking to somebody the other day, I was telling him that it's not the same when he's not around, that I really put a lot of weight on what goes on in our lives together. In the old days, I don't think they called it codependency. I think they called it commitment. Now it has this bad label. I agree that if someone that you're hanging out with is forcing you to do horrifying things against your will, then you are in a bad situation. But if you just love someone so much . . . Years ago when my parents were together and they made all the decisions together and all this stuff, it was a beautiful thing called commitment, love. Now it's codependency. Maybe I am in denial, and if I am I will find out.

The person I profess to be in love with said to me, "I am not in love with you but I love you. Because being in love with you would mean that I could fall out of love with you." And I thought that was really nice. It isn't that I have been robbed again by the English language. It is once again I am not allowed to say that. But I love this man.

What's real love?

I think real love is when you don't want to hurt yourself. I don't know what real love is. I think real love is what I feel when I don't know how to label it. It's just as mysterious as God. There *is* something outrageous about it. I think it's when your heart just glows. I think it's giving someone everything you have because you always get more. If I'm a codependent, so be it. I wave my flag proudly.

Is it important for you to be in a relationship with somebody in the program?

It helps. You need to talk about the steps. You both need to know that you turn things over to God. I don't meet too many people who drink and are spiritual. I have trouble. I am willful. I am exceedingly willful. I want to do things my way all the time and I want them right now. How do you explain that you want to stop being so willful to somebody who is not in the program? That you want to turn your life over to God? How are you going to say, "Oh by the way, I am insane and I am looking for sanity through God?" I know people who are in the program not practicing it. I have learned how to live and let live.

In the beginning I used to want everybody all around me. I was scared and it was nice to go out with people. Now I have broken my support group down to a few really close people. I don't isolate, I insulate. I'm scared. People hurt. They are painful. Maybe I will learn how to trust once more. Maybe when I trust myself, I will be able to trust others. A.A. has taught me so much. I get attracted to things that are not necessarily recovering. I still want to run away. But A.A. tells me so much and teaches me so much and has such a beautiful basic way about it. All those slogans matter so much. They used to be very empty words to me, you know, *"Easy does it, Turn it over, More will be revealed, blab, blab, blab...."* But my feelings have changed since I walked in. My thoughts have changed. I walked into this program a Buddhist freak. I am totally different now. I was searching for answers and now things are being explained. And the more I get into this program, the more I care about myself, the more I want to be with me. I may not always believe it but I've got to say it over and over again. I have a lot of trouble sitting alone and sometimes I feel so isolated, and not just self-isolation but isolated by so many negative people that why would you want to be with them?

Sometimes I wish I was a Barbie with a letter sweater like some sort of freaking cheerleader. I could go to keg parties once a month or fuck guys and it wouldn't matter that they have nothing in them. But it's not that way for me and therefore, you know, I have to respect myself.

Do you have a favorite [A.A.] step?

Three. Three is the ultimate step. *Made a decision to turn our will and lives over to the care of God, as we understood him.* I think without step three you would have nothing. I think without step three it would be hard to do step one. I know they're in order for a reason but there is something about that step three that just *hooks* everything. One thing that doing all those steps in one night has taught me is not to fear speaking commitments. Normally I think I would have flipped. Now I think about how greatly the steps affect my life.

Sometimes I still crave that first naive feeling of getting high, when it was new, and it was fun. I've come close in recovery to relapsing because I have emotionally pulled out and taken my load back. I thank God that I have people who point it out to me. I get to a meeting, because I know me, I know me. I love that life, even though it is hard. There's a slinkiness to it that I have always really enjoyed, and that scares me.

Could you recover with the help of a self-help book?

It's hard to apply something that seems so sterile to a human life. The human life. "Okay, let's use the Step B plan of the Get Your Shit Together Cookbook," you know? But if I read something where somebody is hurting, it makes me think. It really makes me think. I guess that only goes to show you that we only have today. That's cool with me. And if I could believe that every now and then . . . Because I am always pissing on today. With my feet in yesterday and tomorrow.

I've met people in recovery who have cancer, AIDS, *harrowing*

sexual things going on with their parents . . . just terrifying stuff;
death, murder, and they don't pick up. So there has to be something
said for this simple program that is just based on spirituality and
letting go. There has got to be something said for saying that you
are whoever you are, and that you are an alcoholic. There has got
to be something said for a fucking pot of hot coffee. I guess it's all
in the promises, and they come, they come. Just when you think
you have heard them too many times, they are there, and it's wild.
I am just so grateful, so grateful to God that I am in A.A. It's like
you are chosen, you are chosen to survive, you are chosen to learn
new things, so you would be damned if you just turned your face
on that.

December 1990

Sandy

Born and raised in Houston, Texas, she is fifty-two years old. Due to agoraphobia, stress, and trying to relieve some of the tension involved in raising three children alone, she became addicted to Valium. She hit the bottle to ease her panic attacks and took Valium to rid herself of hangovers. She has been married five times. Both of her parents are in A.A. "They have twenty-five years of sobriety. I also have a son in A.A. with four years. A lot of us have died, but a lot of us are alive and sober. My mother is allergic to alcohol. If she took two drinks her face was in her supper— and she's the perfect picture of a Mississippi lady." In the past she has attended both A.A. and Women for Sobriety, but since she went back to school, she only has time for A.A. She has not had a drink since 1971, or a severe anxiety attack. "The worst thing about an attack is the fear of them, that you might have one in front of someone."

I was a periodic drinker. I never drank without getting into trouble. That should have been a signal that there was something wrong. I didn't tolerate alcohol well and I overdrank. When my first marriage broke up, I was suddenly a single mother in a world I didn't know how to deal with. That kicked off big time trouble.

I had to go back to work after nine years. I had three children. My anxiety attacks progressed quite a bit. That's when I obtained the Valium, which really precipitated my drinking. It speeds up an alcohol problem real fast. Within a short period of time, I was in big trouble with Valium and booze. I didn't think that there was a way out of the anxiety.

My parents had already been in A.A. for four years. My excuse for a long time was, "If I ever get as bad as them, I'll quit." Not being aware that I was already in deeper trouble than they had ever been in.

Your drinking was anxiety induced?

Definitely. Alcohol really does calm everything down very quickly. By the time I was twenty-eight, I was diagnosed as an acute, chronic alcoholic. The last few years I drank I was in a fog. It doesn't take very long when you mix alcohol and pills.

I'd get sober for a while and the anxiety attacks would come back, so I'd drink again, or take pills. Unfortunately I was the kind of alcoholic that could function well under the influence. Outwardly. Then I lost my children.

How did you lose them?

One Christmas my ex-husband took them for a visit. He wouldn't give them back. I knew enough that I couldn't argue with him at that point. I knew if I went and got the law, they would probably be on his side. Then my mother took them. I never went to court. I kept threatening to, but I never did. I started getting children back after three years of sobriety. My mother called me out of the clear blue and said, "Come get the oldest one; I can't stand him." My youngest son called about nine months later and said come get him, and about then my daughter called and said come get her. I ended up raising my friend's daughter.

Do many women get sober in Women for Sobriety?

We have a lot of women who have gotten sober in Women for Sobriety and haven't done anything else. I think we need alternatives to the twelve-step format. I like the twelve-step format immensely. It's helped a lot of people, but there are some women, particularly your agoraphobics, that need more. I didn't know what agoraphobic meant, but I was one back yonder.

Were you ever housebound?

No, I just had trouble leaving the house. I got claustrophobia in the car. I had a real hard time even after I sobered up, for a couple of years. I would sit outside of the grocery store in the car with the sweats, for half an hour before I could go in and buy groceries. Some of it was fear of buying booze instead of groceries because I hadn't bought groceries without buying booze for so long. A lot of it was fear of people and crowds. I had a lot of trouble with meetings. Before I got sober, I was having anxiety attacks to the point of hyperventilating.

I used to start out with real short breaths, like I couldn't quite get my breath. Like the start of an asthma attack but not quite. I'm an asthmatic as well. The panic I was feeling was like the asthma, but it was more of a smothery feeling. I was scared out of my wits but I couldn't have told you why—I had no earthly idea. I didn't know for years what was going on. I went to a doctor. He said it was just anxiety. This was in the sixties. He suggested I try relaxation meditation. I wasn't at an emotional place in my life to pay attention to meditation. He suggested that my life was not well-rounded enough and I needed more hobbies. I was a single mother with a house full of children and a lot of responsibility and took it entirely too seriously. But nothing really worked and I ended up with Valium and Elavil, which is an antidepressant.

Nobody had the time for agoraphobia back then, or they didn't want to take it. I didn't have the money for counseling. I'm an Episcopalian, and I saw a priest. I got some counseling through my church, but it wasn't enough. The medication helped to some extent. No one asked me if I had a bottle problem.

I don't know what the chemistry is, but alcohol can really aggravate the heck out of hysteria or panic. Especially coming off alcohol the next day. Rather than a hangover you have what I used to call grand mal panic attacks. That's how I got into medication. It progressed to the point where I could not get it calmed down or stopped. I was feeling like I was going to smother and not get my breath. The next stage was shaking all over and sweating. Sometimes the next stage would be going into full-blown hyperventilation. I fell down several times at work. One time my boss got so concerned he took me to the emergency room. The doctor showed me how to breathe into a brown bag. It was awful, just awful.

Does breathing into a paper bag help?

Oh, yeah, it will stop it and it will keep you from falling out.

What do you mean by falling out—fainting?

Almost like fainting, yes. Once or twice I lost consciousness. I understand it's very common for people under a lot of stress. It never was a problem when I was sober. I had some problems the first couple of years but it never went into hyperventilation. I had the shaking and the sweating, to where I would have to take a shower and change my clothes. It never progressed to hyperventilating after I got sober. I haven't had an attack in years and years.

I've been through a lot of counseling. That's really important. I think it would have taken forever to get over the panic attacks without outside help. The A.A. program isn't enough; it isn't designed for that type of anxiety. The program is there to help you get your life turned around and make a new start. But for people with problems, you are going to have to go outside.

As time went on, particularly with counseling and learning to be in new situations, a counselor helped me to understand that I needed to walk into rooms full of people, whether I knew them or not, and it would be okay.

How did you decide you wanted to get sober?

I was driving in the car, and out of the clear blue sky I had a panic attack. I was on a country road on the way to my sister's house and I had to get out and walk around. I would still like to say it was God speaking to me. I really didn't know what it was, but all of a sudden I was fully aware of the fact that if I didn't do something I wasn't going to live for very long.

I had been drinking for seven or eight years on a consistent basis. I was also taking about 100 mg. a day of Valium and I don't know how much Elavil, plus sleeping pills. I was drinking about a fifth of Jack Daniels a day, or whatever else I could get. I had a nurse tell me that I had toxic poisoning from the combination of chemicals and booze. I had enough sense about me at the time to be fully aware that my emotions were dying. My emotions were blocked with all the booze and medications. I was a walking zombie. I had been in and out of A.A. for a couple of years, but I never did stop drinking.

At the time, I lived approximately thirteen miles from Rusk State Hospital. When I got out to my sister's house that day, I asked her to take me to the hospital. She didn't think I was serious. She was horrified at the idea of a family member being at a state hospital. I told her that I would call the sheriff's department if she wouldn't take me. I was well aware that they would love to get me off the streets. I already had one DWI.

The next morning she realized that I was dead serious. She packed me up in her little Dodge van that she had at the time and drove me the thirteen miles to Rusk.

At that time they had a couple of different programs you could sign up for. They had one of the best alcohol programs in the state. I asked them not to release me until the doctor thought I was ready to leave. You can sign yourself in and you can sign yourself out. But I told them not to release me, regardless of what I said and did, until the doctor thought I was ready to leave. I ended up staying there for seven weeks.

It was eighteen days of DTs and convulsions, because of all of the crap I had been taking. I didn't know what they were going to do. One of the reasons I hadn't gone before was because I had heard some of the tales about the shock treatments that were done on alcoholics in the fifties. This was in April of '71 and they had passed some sort of deal stating that shock treatments would not be used except for extenuating circumstances. They would not be used without the patient's consent unless it was someone who was totally uncontrollable. I wasn't in a condition to need shock treatment for any reason, but I had it in my mind for several years that that is what they do to alcoholics. They explained to me that they had other things that worked better, including therapy and one-on-one counseling.

The program was fantastic. I had a couple of group meetings a day, and individual counseling every day. When I had been there a couple of weeks, I went to occupational therapy and vocational testing. The physical testing was the best I have had in my entire life. From top to bottom, all shots were brought up to date, even tetanus shots, like what kids get.

Was the panic addressed?

Oh yes. They didn't know as much about it then, but they were well aware of the problem. It was a real big thing going through withdrawal. I didn't like mixing with people. I didn't like the groups for that reason. It was very difficult to learn to talk in front of a room full of people. I was unaware that I had a lot of anger. I knew I was depressed, severely depressed. One counselor really got me in touch with my anger in a group one day. I left the group and said I wasn't going to go back, which is kind of dumb when you're shut up in a state hospital. In a couple of days I began to realize a lot of the things that were said were true. It was mostly fear behind the panic attacks. You know it doesn't take but three or four fears that are not dealt with, and the next thing you know you don't want to leave the house.

It doesn't have to start out being a big fear. It starts out having fear of getting on a bus or driving across town. I had fears of walking into A.A. meetings full of people I didn't know. If I had allowed that to build without dealing with it, it would have gotten worse. My sponsor would take me to a meeting and he would sit in the car until I got inside, then he would come in. If I was in trouble, he could tell by my expression. If I was okay, he went about his business in the room with other people. I couldn't do it alone. The day came when I had to drag myself to a meeting and go in by myself. I shook through the whole thing and I couldn't talk, but I did go.

It was a real gradual process. I had to learn that nobody was going to bite me. In spite of my fears of a panic attack it was not going to happen. I think one of the worst things that happens to people with panic attacks is the fear of them. You get to where you're afraid to go places because you don't want to have an attack in front of people.

Sometimes I would walk around to get some fresh air and try to breathe normally. I carried my little paper bag with me for a long time. I didn't have to use it as it turned out. I thought I was going to have to one time, the first time I went grocery shopping totally alone and sober. I had been sober nearly two years by then. I sat outside in the car for about an hour and it was cold. February, cold, cold, cold and I was sweating so bad I had to get out of the car and walk around. I finally made it inside that store and I just kept concentrating on going up and down the aisles and getting my groceries. By the time I left, I was fine. But I was scared out of my wits. One of the things I learned is that if I just keep doing the things that I have to do the symptoms would go away. My fears of the symptoms aggravated it.

So you had to trust.

Oh, you're not kidding. Do what you have to do, the old A.A. thing, I guess, of putting one foot in front of the other. Whatever is supposed to happen will.

Do you think cutting down on caffeine decreases the frequency of panic attacks?

Definitely, and chocolate too. I used to be a chocoholic first class. I don't make fudge anymore. The last time I made a great big thing of fudge, five or six years ago, I ended up eating the whole plate, it looked so good. I woke up the next day, not only with the shakes but very depressed. I don't make fudge anymore and I don't buy chocolate anymore because I think it just aggravates it. I think a lot of preservatives might aggravate it also, so I use a lot of frozen vegetables because most of those don't have very many preservatives. I stick to fresh fruits. I have learned to read labels and I stick with a low fat diet—a lot of fish, chicken, turkey, vegetables and fruits.

How did you get interested in Women for Sobriety after being in A.A.?

I had moved here a little over eight years ago, due to a divorce. I was making a lot of living adjustments. I was past forty and for the first time in my entire life was living alone. Before, I had either a husband or a houseful of children. The last child left home and went into the navy four months after I moved here. I do have a doberman dog, but I had no people for the first time. I read an ad in the downtown newspaper about groups for women working on sobriety and another way to live, or something. Someone from Women for Sobriety put those ads in the paper. I called the number and the lady immediately called me back. She said that they had several groups going and that it was all women. They pretty much just stuck to women's issues for sobriety. They dealt with middle-aged women with fears of living alone and starting a new life. At the time, I was living on the north side of town. I started going out to some meetings and Cindy, the moderator, was wonderful. She was one of those gorgeous mother images. She was standing in the doorway with her arms open. I needed that at that point. She's a very loving and giving, fantastic female.

In those groups I was able to share my fears of silly stuff . . . every pot I owned was humongous because I raised a houseful of teenagers. I was by myself so I gave away all my big pots, with the exception of a couple. There were so many itty bitty problems; I couldn't see the solutions to any of them. I didn't know how to cook for a single person. I had leftovers running out of my ears so I would end up snacking instead of cooking. I started reading books. One book suggested learning to cook smaller portions and explained how to snip recipes, and how to simplify your meals. Some of it was really simple stuff, I just couldn't see a simple answer. I had too many things in my head bothering me.

I didn't think that I could go anywhere unless someone was with me. I hadn't been anywhere alone in thirty years. I always had a husband or kids.

The W.F.S. group helped me to see that I needed to learn to start making some moves for myself—that I could go to a movie for instance. I could go to a Saturday matinee, I didn't have to go at night. I was afraid of going and coming out at night. A lot of it was fears of going places alone. What the hell was I going to do with all of this time since I was alone? I overdid it for a couple of years with a lot of handwork, crocheting and macrame. I took on a second job at a grocery store. I didn't really need the money that bad, but it came in handy. Without the group's support it would have definitely been difficult.

So you were going to A.A. and Women for Sobriety and you really liked doing both?

Definitely. I miss Women for Sobriety partly because of the women's discussions. There are a lot of issues in sobriety that are very definitely, whether people like it or not, female oriented. Women are more dependent. I think we can learn not to be, but basically society teaches us to be. We have different viewpoints, and we come at most situations with our emotions. Men go at them more with their heads. I think most of us, before sobriety, put more emphasis on male friendships and have a lack in the department of female friendships. I had to learn how to make female friends. Learning to share the good things, not just the bad things.

One of my biggest conflicts with W.F.S. is Jean's [Kirkpatrick] feeling that A A is for men. That is hogwash. Real hogwash. I do think there is a real big need for women's groups but A.A. has a lot of women's groups.

Isn't it easier for a man to get up and say, I slept with all these women, than for a woman to get up and say, I slept with all these men?

Women still need to learn to say those things if they are going to be cleared. I have been married five times, for instance. I had a lot of relationship problems. If I didn't like something, I left. Now, in a mixed A.A. meeting, sometimes men take that to mean I have a sex problem. They don't see that I have a relationship problem. I had to learn to battle a lot of people and I learned not to share in some meetings. One problem alcoholics have is relationships. We don't know how to cope with them. If we did we wouldn't be in A.A. or any other alcoholic programs. Alcoholics are charming and witty. They're the most intelligent people on God's green earth, but they have zero coping skills. People with zero coping skills can either sleep around or they can marry all of them. I married them.

Did you get married after you got sober?

Oh, yes. The last one I married I suspect was an antisocial personality disorder.

Are you married now?

No, ma'am. I have been single for over eight years and I love it.
I learned to deal with that addiction. I've gone back to school. I'm
trying to finish an associate in mental health. In January I'm going
to find out if I can transfer to Our Lady of the Lake and I am going
for a bachelor's in human resources. I'm almost ready to take my
Texas test for alcohol and drug abuse counseling.

So your goal is to be a counselor?

Of some sort. I would love to teach. I am fifty-two and a half and
sick of what I'm doing. It's real high pressure. It's good money and
pays for school, but I can't do it forever. I wrote to social security
a couple of years ago to see what my retirement benefits would be
at sixty-two and at sixty-five. It's only going to be about $575 a
month. I can't live on that. I couldn't live on it today. I'm going for
my master's so I can teach at the junior college level part-time, and
make enough money.

*What would you say to a woman who said she was afraid to give up alcohol
or drugs because of panic attacks?*

That is a sorry excuse. That's a sorry excuse not to get clean. I
understand there is a real viable fear, but there are too many people
in the field that know how to deal with anxiety today. There weren't
when I sobered up. I did it the *hard* way. I don't know anyone today
that doesn't know how to deal with panic attacks and fears. They
have to deal with some of their own or they're never going to get
through the Texas test. I don't know of any fear you cannot overcome
if you're willing to go through real good treatment. There are a lot
of good outpatient treatments now. You don't have to go into the
hospital if you don't want. Even a good social worker can help. You
don't have to have high price psychiatry. Our problems are day-to-
day issues, of women alone, and women alone with children. There's
plenty of help available.

December 1990

Marion

The sixty-two-year-old woman who opens the door of her brownstone to me in Charlestown, Massachusetts, is disarming. She is small, five feet three, yet even before she speaks I sense a woman with huge amounts of physical and emotional strength. She has fine features, eyebrows so delicate they look finely etched or painted. But there is nothing false about her. Clear and blue, her eyes have taken things in and sorted them out. She talks and thinks, remembers and laughs, and sometimes she looks sad. Her husband, Jim, is an attorney and a recovering alcoholic. They met in Alcoholics Anonymous. Their house is beautiful, an accurate reflection of the people who live in it. Carefully chosen and well-cared-for antiques, six shelves of cookbooks in the kitchen—there are stories connected to every possession. She has been married to Jim for fourteen years. Jim is not home but one gets a sense of him. "Jim made that clock," she points out, "and that table over there, he made it when he was a boy." In 1983 Marion graduated from Harvard Divinity School. She has been sober since 1975.

I really didn't start drinking until I was in my late teens. I had started college and I was on a date with a fellow who had just come back from World War II. He had come to the college I was going to. He asked me out and when we went out for dinner he asked me what I wanted to drink. I looked at him rather blankly and he said, "I'll decide for you." So he got me a Pink Lady. And I think how far I've progressed from that innocuous lady's drink.

When I was a little girl my father didn't drink very much. He'd come home from work and he'd be happy and he was fun to be with. I was Daddy's girl. As I got to be a teenager, his drinking increased, and it reached the point where my mother would sit in the window to watch to see him come home from work. The longer it took, the more irritated she would get and I'd say, "Please, God, don't let there be a fight." Of course the minute she opened the door she'd say something to him like, "Well, where have you been?" And World War III would start. I'd go up to my room and turn on my radio to drown out the noise.

My parents had "his and hers" kids. My brother was totally my mother's kid so I had little contact with my mother. The nurturing I really should have gotten from her I didn't get. I got a lot of other things. I got a sense of independence, a sense of having to stand on my own two feet, and being strong. I got all As in school. I can remember five girls who lived next door—an Irish family. They were beautiful. I can remember my mother talking about how pretty they were. I said to her, "Am I pretty?" and she said, "No, but you'll do." It was that kind of lack of support that really made me feel inadequate.

I married early, in my sophomore year of college. I had started dating a man who was ten years older than I was. My parents didn't approve of him. I managed to get pregnant. I married him because that was the thing to do, and within a few months I knew that it wasn't right. I realize now that one of the things I wanted to do was get out of my parents' house.

So I started out and of course my house was going to be perfect and different from my parents' house. We had our little boy, and my husband started running around. I wouldn't admit there was anything wrong. I certainly wasn't going to let my parents know that they had been right.

We had a nice home. We had another little boy six years later and bought a big house. Then the entertaining began. My husband was very, very insecure and didn't feel like he was worth anything. His way of building himself up was to tear me down. Every day I heard that if it wasn't for him, I'd be nothing. I stayed in that marriage for fourteen years.

It's hard to know whether or not to cave in and be what men want us to be.

I think you can only cave in and be what they want you to be if you're willing to sell your soul. And that's what I did for the fourteen years I was in that marriage. The verbal abuse became terrible. He would yell at night when he got home. On the outside he was charming and people thought he was wonderful, but they didn't see what I saw. His mother once said to him, "You're lucky to have a woman like her, she's a big help to you." And I thought to myself, "Oh, I'm gonna get it tonight." And sure enough . . . he just couldn't handle that. All of this fed those feelings of inadequacy that I already had.

I began to find out that if I had a couple of drinks, I'd feel okay about myself. I didn't feel so stupid. I didn't feel like I had two left feet when I was going to dance, so I drank at parties. I always drank with fear, because I never ever wanted to be drunk. My mother used to drink with my father on the weekends. She'd say, "I have to do this in order to stand him." I could accept my father's alcoholism, but I couldn't accept my mother's. I'm not even sure that she was alcoholic, but it was disgusting. She was disgusting. Mothers don't *do* that. I know now that that's a lot of the programming that we got as young women growing up. Women are always ladies and they always do everything just right. They're the backbone of the home, the angel of the hearth and all that nonsense that we learned. She once said, "You could forgive him anything but you could never forgive me." And she was absolutely right. Absolutely right. That's exactly the way I felt. So whenever I drank, I always drank with a dose of guilt. If anyone had ever said to me then that I would become alcoholic I'd say, "Don't be ridiculous, I don't drink like my father. I don't stop at bars on my way home from work. I just do this when we entertain."

This entertaining got to be every night. I got to the point where I could tell him off once in a while, but I usually paid for it. One night we were at a party that started in the afternoon and went 'til around eleven, and the verbal abuse became physical. And with that I left. I just took the two kids and some clothes and put them in the car.

The last thing he did was to throw one of those big Belgian blocks they pave the streets with in Boston, through the back window of the car.

I went to my parents' and asked if we could stay for a couple of days until I could find a place to live and their reaction was, "How could you do this to us? There's never been a divorce in this family. This is disgusting. You should go back to him." But I didn't. I found a little three-room apartment.

I started dating another fellow, named Bill, and he drank a lot.
He was a friend from the party crowd we'd been involved with and
he was going through a divorce, too. Bill and I started going out.
We'd have a couple of martinis before dinner. I was not comfortable
with that. In the beginning when I was alone with the kids I hadn't
been drinking. I was beginning to feel good about myself. When I
started drinking again, I had some more of that guilt.

One night Bill called me at about 3 A.M. and said there were snakes
crawling around his room. I thought he must be crazy. I had no idea
of alcoholism. Nobody did in those days. This was in 1960, and
nobody really talked about it or knew anything about it. I'd read an
article in, I think it was *The Saturday Evening Post*, on alcoholism
and I wondered if that's what he had. I didn't hear from him for a
week and I thought I had done something wrong. Naturally I thought
that. Then he called me and told me he'd been going to A.A. meetings
and that he would still like to see me but he had to go to these
meetings and would I go with him. I did, and right from the beginning I *loved* A.A. I loved the people and the caring and everything
about it. They were so happy and that was really what came through
to me, the happiness. There were people who'd been in trouble and
they were laughing. I was in my early thirties.

I stopped drinking when he did. I went to meetings and at first I
started listening for him; then I really began listening for myself. I
was having a glass of wine at night to put me to sleep. I had it hidden
at the back of the refrigerator so if Bill opened it he wouldn't see it.
And then I heard people talk about hiding bottles. I didn't see anything alcoholic about that, I did it. But somebody pointed out to me
that there were not degrees of alcoholism, just degrees of trouble.
And at that point I accepted the fact that I was alcoholic.

Bill and I were married. Three years to the day we were married,
he died of cancer. He had found out earlier that year and it was a
very tough year. I did everything for Bill except give him his shots.

A year later a friend of mine had an art exhibit, an opening, in
Hingham. And I met another man, his name was John. He was very
attractive and charming. Obviously he'd been drinking. He admitted
he was an alcoholic. He drank himself out of his law practice. He
owned a bar called The Club Car. I got mixed up with him and I
was going to straighten him out. I knew he drank too much, but I
thought if things get out of hand I'd take him to A.A. and he'd be
all right.

He said, "If you marry me, Marion, it will be the worst thing you
ever did in your life." And he was absolutely right. I married him.
It was a drunken wedding. I was drinking to keep up with him, not
knowing that it takes half as much for a woman to get drunk as it
does for a man.

It was a wild round of parties from then on. I decided to sell my
house and I bought a house that I couldn't afford with the idea that
John would be contributing to it. I gave him money to set himself
up with a law practice and he drank himself out of that. He did not
contribute to the house so we started getting behind in the payments.
John would be passed out on the chair so I'd make myself a couple
of drinks to forget it or I'd have to go and get him at The Club Car;
he couldn't drive home.

My youngest son, Ronnie, was still home. When Bill died, Rick
went into the Marine Corps and then to Vietnam. There was a lot
going on.

It was just Ronnie and me when I met John. Things got really
horrible down in Hingham. I went to the doctor and told him I was
very nervous. Naturally I was nervous. I was drinking every night.
The doctor gave me some Valium for my nerves, and I thought that
was a good idea. I knew from A.A. not to drink and take the pills,
so if I was going to drink I simply didn't take the pills.

A party starting on Saturday ended up at our house on Sunday.
At two in the afternoon John decided to have a steak dinner and I
said, "You're out of your mind. I can't cook. I'm stiff." and he said,
"I'll cook." And I tried to explain that we needed salad and dessert.
But he was so insistent that I ended up taking the whole bottle of
Valium. I was going to show him that I could not cook a steak
dinner. I told him, "Now I took this whole bottle of pills and I can't
cook dinner." Somebody gave me some coffee. John said, "Well, if
she can't cook we'll all go down to The Club Car and have dinner."
My son Ronnie took me to the Norwood hospital.

I had on a bright green velour top that I just loved and a pair of
white pants. I had spilled coffee all over the front of my pants which
left a big brown stain. God, I was just a mess and I was sick inside.
After that I kept saying to myself, "You know, Marion, there's a
better way to live." I didn't want to go through another divorce.
Here I'd been married three times and I couldn't admit to another
failure. The next day, coming home from work, I had a spiritual
experience, and I truly believe that we all have a spiritual experience

that starts us on this road. This was the moment when I knew that when I got home John was going to be drunk and that I was an alcoholic and needed to go to A.A. Not for husbands. But for me.

I made up my mind that I was going to A.A. After work I just changed my clothes and I went off to a meeting. And for the next two months we didn't say one word to each other. At meetings I was complaining because John was taking my money and writing checks to The Club Car, and so someone in A.A. said, "Don't put money in that account. Open up another one in your name." So I did. I told him and the next morning he confronted me. We had a conversation. He said, "If you feel that way about the money I want a separation." And I said, "You've got it."

Monday morning on my way to work I said, "Okay, God, if you want me to move out of this house you're going to have to tell me where to go because I don't know what to do." And about five miles down the road I passed a house that had a For Rent sign on it. I rented it. And that was the beginning of a real change. I moved out of the house and left John enough stuff to exist until the bank took it.

I got really wrapped up in A.A. I met a fellow the first night I went and asked him to be my sponsor until I could find a woman. And so he did and we became very close. That was Jim. Then I *knew* I needed a woman. I needed to get some distance. I did find a woman, and it was a lot of tough A.A. I started using her for a sponsor and that was better because there were times when I was getting a pat on the back when I needed a kick in the ass.

I continued seeing Jim. I had my first anniversary. It was held at an open meeting and everyone I knew was there. It was just a wonderful meeting. Everyone was so glad I was sober. Life was good. Jim and I were married. Jim knew I loved school, and he said, "Why don't you go back?" and I did. I went to the University of New Hampshire and got a degree in philosophy with a minor in religion. I loved school. And then Jim said, "Why don't you go to graduate school? Why don't you go to divinity school, because that's what you've been studying. Go to Harvard." I applied and I was accepted. I graduated in 1987. I was sixty.

What was that like?

It was hard. It was fun. It's not as close a community as you'd expect. There were a lot of lesbians, not very many gays. There were as many women as there were men. There were as many older people as younger people. So, it was an eclectic community. There's a lot of emphasis at Harvard on women's liberation.

When I started divinity school, we moved to Boston and bought this house. I also had a job going all over the country teaching drug and alcohol education. I tried, whenever I could, to get to meetings out of town. This is something that Jim and I have always done. One of the first things he taught me was that if I was going to A.A. I'd better learn to make it fun or I wouldn't keep it up. And so we would do things like drive out of town and have dinner and go to a meeting.

I've been to meetings from Maine to Panama. I've been to meetings where I couldn't understand the language. It's like you don't know the words but you can hear the music. And so it was wonderful.

I taught for FCD* for a couple of years. I really got the sense that you can talk to these kids till you're deaf, dumb, and blind, but if you don't get to the parents you're not going to get anywhere. At that point I graduated from Harvard, and I thought, "Now what am I going to do?" Because I knew I didn't want to continue what I was doing. I didn't feel it was enough. People kept saying to me, "Are you going to be a minister?" and I said, "No."

I said, "Well, God will show me what I need to do when it's time to do it." I graduated on Thursday and on Friday my boss from FCD called and asked if I would be the director of development. And I said, "I'll give it a try." So I did that for a year. And I didn't really like it. I don't like development work. I don't like asking people for money. I don't mind writing the proposals, but going and playing footsie and trying to get something from them is not my cup of tea. And so I told him I didn't want to do that anymore, I wanted to go back to teaching. FCD has mostly recovering people in it, and it's just like a dysfunctional family. And the control issues of "I want you to do this. . . . " Finally I said, "Enough of this."

People were saying to me, "Why don't you do it on your own? You can go teach. You don't need FCD to teach." And I said, "That's ridiculous, I'm sixty years old. Why would I want to start a business at this point? I'm ready to retire." I got this from Jim and from three other friends. I firmly believe that when you start getting messages

Freedom from Chemical Dependency.

from more than one place—like when one person says you really
ought to read this book and then three others say it too, I go buy
the book. I was still iffy and then another woman who used to work
for FCD called and said, "I would like to start doing this, will you
do it with me?" And I said, "Okay God, I've got the message. This
is probably what I'm supposed to be doing next."

So we started a little company using both of our last names. A
woman from University Bank decided that she wanted to do things
like alcohol education in the Brookline schools. They have a lot of
business there. And so for the last three years we've done all the
alcohol and drug education. I'd realized that I'd really rather teach
adults. I met a fellow who's the head of the Boston EAP,* and he
wanted to start concentrating on women, because he felt that women
were falling through the cracks. Only eight percent of the people in
his program were women. We know that women represent *at least*
thirty-eight percent of alcoholics.

I started doing a lot of teaching for him. The business isn't really
making any money but we're able to pay for advertising. We've done
some good work. My partner Joannie's been doing all the work in
the Brookline schools. Working with managers and supervisors, en-
couraging them to get these women into treatment, to recognize the
early warning signs, to talk to their women about the fact it's okay
to be an alcoholic. And then getting the employer to say, "We want
you in treatment, we'll pay for it, and we want you back as a good
productive worker."

What happens is the minute an employer mentions drugs and
alcohol to a woman—a man will bluster and say, "I don't need that,
I'm perfectly fine"; the woman won't. But the next day she'll call
in and say, "I'm not going to work here anymore. I was planning
to quit anyway...." What I've been pointing out to them is this
might be the only chance for the woman to get sober, and that if
they would just spend that little bit of extra time to get the woman
into treatment, they would end up with a better employee. They'd
also end up with somebody in place who can then recognize a drug
and alcohol problem in other workers and they'll have a built-in
support system to help them.

I've been talking to employers about the fact that the work place
is like another family. There are codependency issues. Employees

Employee assistance program.

who have a drinking problem blame other people. Everyone is wondering, "Is she going to come in today?" It makes their own jobs harder.

When did you go from being Daddy's girl to caring so much about women?

I think it started at divinity school because there was so much emphasis on feminism. And the lesbians are rabid. It's unfortunate, because they do themselves a lot of harm.

When I was at divinity school I realized that no one knew anything about alcoholism. So every paper I wrote, everything that I did, centered on alcoholism. I took a course in anthropology and used A.A. as the community that I studied. I took a course that had to do with the problems women ministers have. And minorities also. I would ask questions. The lesbians were saying, "People don't understand, they don't understand anything about us." And I said, "Well, tell me," and they said, "Well, you wouldn't understand." I went home. It was really bothering me. You get the same thing from the blacks. "If you aren't a part of our culture, you just don't understand." And I realized the same was true with alcoholism. So I wrote a paper on alcoholism.

I went in the next day and I said, "I'd like to read this. I'm going to get emotional about it and if I read it I won't explode." But basically what I said was, "I would like you to listen to me, I need you to tell me *what* I wouldn't understand. *Tell* me how you feel. Help me to understand because at some point when I'm working with alcoholics I'm going to run into somebody who is black, or who is a lesbian, and I want to be able to help them. I want you to listen to me because I can *guarantee* that you're going to run into some alcoholics and maybe if you've known me and know how I think and how I've felt, you'll have a better understanding of who they are." It really opened the class up. It was something that they hadn't thought of.

This is something that I find with a lot of ministers. They know nothing about alcoholism, yet they're the people, next to the doctors, who will come in contact with it the most. Another thing I've done, with doctors, is role playing. I teach them how to confront an alcoholic; a woman comes in and is complaining of stomach pains and he realizes that she's drinking. How does he or she confront this? It's amazing; they just don't know. One young woman said, "How much alcohol do you use?" and I found after fifteen years of sobriety I'm going "Eeeeh! Get me away from this woman." I pointed that out to the others who were watching the role play. I said, "How much do you drink?" It's a simple question. Don't put it in such an awkward light because you push people away.

Is there anything else?

The basic message is that A.A. works but it's not a cure-all. And that's important because I know that judges and lawyers, doctors and ministers, and police all say, "Go to A.A., that's going to fix everything." A.A. doesn't fix everything. It helps you to get sober so that you can grow and then you can fix everything. People don't grow unless they start working on the steps. The spiritual part of the program is vital.

I was always searching for the Higher Power that was right for me, the religion that was right for me. That's one of the reasons why I didn't get a masters in divinity. I didn't want to take any church polity because I didn't believe in any of them.

The first course that I took at divinity school was a course in spirituality. It was fantastic. The professor was wonderful. The last course I took was on process theology, which is a new way of looking at religion. It's based on Whitehead's philosophy. Everything is energy and everything is divided into moments, rather than everything is divided into atoms and molecules. It ties in with the A.A. philosophy. I wrote my final paper on that, that A.A. was in fact a vehicle for expressing process theology.

It's amazing the way things have happened. In my life I've learned to *Let Go and Let God* because God's visions—No, I hate to use those kinds of terms. My God is not a him or a her or an it, and process theology taught me that. They call God creative transformation; that God is and it's the new thing that comes into each moment of our existence. Everything is in process and God is something new that comes in and prevents things from running down. There's some force that is guiding us if we allow ourselves to be guided. If I align myself with God's will, and that uses those terms in a way that I don't like . . . if I align myself with this force then my life becomes a lot more than what I could envision for it. Because my vision is too small.

March 1990

Part Five

Self-Worth

I'm often asked what it's like being married
to a genius. The question used to please
me—as an affirmation of my place, of my
counting for something (if only through
marriage) in the only world that counted for
anything.

> —Rebecca Goldstein,
> *The Mind-Body Problem*

Jean Kirkpatrick

Jean Kirkpatrick was born in 1923. In 1971 she put down her last drink. In 1976 she wrote some personal affirmations to get her through the day, and thus Women for Sobriety was inadvertently founded. She was fifty-three when she decided it was a matter of survival—she wasn't getting sober through A.A., and alcohol was killing her. Jean's program was not private for very long. United Press International surfaced with a press release about Women for Sobriety and 2,000 letters from women who had complaints about A.A. appeared on her doorstep. A quiet revolution began. There are over 30,000 women who belong to Women for Sobriety. Groups are scattered all over the country.

I was in A.A. for about three years. And then in the fifties, I started drinking again and drank for about thirteen more years. Of course, I got very ill. I was in and out of hospitals. I attempted suicide several times and went back to A.A., but could not make it work. There was nothing about it that was appealing anymore. I don't know why, but everything about it seemed wrong to me. I went to meetings and I felt very negative, I felt very depressed. I'd come out of a meeting and I'd want a drink, so quite obviously that was not my way to sobriety.

I started to ask myself why, why was I drinking? What was the basis of it? I would have two or three days of sobriety. Then I'd start drinking again. I asked myself what had happened to make me start drinking again, and I found that the basis of it was that I was feeling very sorry for myself. I felt like nobody loved me, totally alienated from the world.

I thought if those were my feelings, and if those feelings made me drink, maybe I could start an individual program for myself by which I might reverse them. It seemed that the basis for getting well for me, and for women, was having good feelings about myself. That's the way I started.

Do you believe alcoholism is a disease?

I believe there must be something in you, because if I look back to when I first started drinking, I was an alcoholic almost from the very beginning. I drank more than anybody else. That was in my freshman year of college.

People ask me what the difference is between heavy drinkers and alcoholics. I try to describe the physical pain and I don't get too far.

I think the difference is there's a compulsive craving that's a physical craving. But there are now enough studies to back this up. People who are alcoholics do handle alcohol, physiologically, quite differently from others. So I think what's more interesting is that in a third of all alcoholics it's a gene factor.

It's a very difficult thing to pin down and it's even more difficult for the public because it's a social amenity, as opposed to, say, other drug addictions. When people come into your home the first thing you say is, "Will you have a drink?" and that means alcohol, not iced tea. It's a part of our culture. You don't hear people say, "Will you have a form of crack?"

That's why it's so difficult for the general public to accept it as a disease.

How did you start Women for Sobriety?

I started realizing that I needed to have some good feelings about myself. I wrote things down. Every day I'd write affirmations and read them and pretty soon I was starting to build some sobriety.

About a year or two later I was in my fifties and I couldn't get a job. I was a woman. I was overtrained. I had a Ph.D. in sociology. I was overage and an alcoholic. Finally I thought, "Gee whiz, maybe some other women might have problems with A.A.," never realizing how many there were. I just thought there were a few. Of course since that time, 1976, our files are bulging. We have over thirty thousand women who have written.

Is there a common complaint about A.A.?

In A.A. you turn yourself over, and as women have been forced to turn themselves over to their fathers, husbands, to everyone, I think this is just the last straw. I think what our program tries to do is to give women some empowerment. We need to have control of our lives; we need to have control of ourselves. Plus in A.A. the basis is humility. What woman that you know of needs more humility?

I also don't think any program can be totally successful if it's built on threats: "If you don't attend you'll relapse, medication is always bad. . . . " And that's what it is. We have women, and I feel so sorry about this, women who go to A.A. and have trouble with the program, and what they get is, "If you work this program right you won't want anything else." And so that means that the fault lies with you, not with the program; the fault is yours.

I think it leaves the thinking person very confused. I think sometimes they say, "Don't think, just do." That saying "Keep it simple, stupid"* is just the pits.

Is it harder for intelligent people?

Yes. We want to know why it works or why it doesn't work, and why are we feeling this. We try to use an intelligent approach to understanding our illness. I think it's unfortunate when programs say, "Don't ask any questions. Just do this and it will all work out."

I think it's unconscionable that A.A. won't recognize any other program. What that does is make the recovered person feel she is

*An A.A. slogan.

flawed if she doesn't get A.A. That just adds another burden to the person who's trying to recover. And prepare yourself for flack. I mean I have been bucking the system since 1974 when I did my first interview with UPI, which appeared in 160 papers. I got a nasty letter from A.A. headquarters in New York, because I said I had been a member of A.A. and no longer was. They wrote and said to keep quiet. I sent a blistering letter back. They have no right to tell me who I am, or what to say.

They can't shut you up. But isn't it terrible to think that there's this big organization that has to be so petty? It's a miracle that we have been able to survive, because all treatment facilities, all 7,000 of them in this country, are based on A.A.

Is it financial? A.A. is free.

That's a part of it, although Women for Sobriety is also free. We suggest a two-dollar donation. A.A. often asks for a "silent" donation. The other part of it is almost everybody that owns a treatment facility or is on the board of directors is a male recovered alcoholic from A.A. Now when I used to be on the road doing seminars on Women for Sobriety, the women who attended were therapists and counselors from treatment facilities. When I outlined what Women for Sobriety did, that the basic premise was to build self-confidence and security and empowerment, all the therapists and women would sit there and say, "This is it. This is exactly what the women in our treatment center need." So they'd take all these papers back to their director, who was a male. And he'd nix it right there because it wasn't A.A. I've been doing this now for fifteen years and we're in about twenty treatment facilities.

So there is a choice in some treatment facilities.

A few, yes, but can you imagine, after all these years, W.F.S. is in just a few. It's a disgrace.

I've met women who have drifted out of A.A. and they all say, "I don't want to put A.A. down because they do marvelous work."

The letters I've gotten are exactly like that. They'll say "Well, I'm so interested in Women for Sobriety. I believe this is the program I

really want. Now I'm not trying to say anything against A.A.—but
. . ." They always have to put in that disclaimer.

Why?

Because of the guilt A.A. has created. If you leave their program
you are flawed, not the program. Alcoholics already have over-
whelming guilt feelings and to have this additional guilt feeling hung
on them by A.A. . . .
They make everybody get off all medications but, you see, they
cover themselves: it's nowhere in writing. It's not anywhere in the
traditions. Yet you go to any group and they'll immediately tell you
that you've got to get off all medications which is really playing with
fire, particularly for hypertensives or diabetics. If you put this in a
book, they'll deny it. But the groups do it. In A.A. literature from
general service, they say that they respect other programs, but in
actual practice that's not true.

I've gotten some great stories from women in A.A.

Well, that's fine. Your point of view should be that there are some
who have successfully used A.A. I have never been able to understand—most of the women I meet are generally feminists—I have
never been able to understand how in the hell you can be a feminist
and be a died-in-the-wool A.A. woman. I don't understand how
you can resolve the conflict between seeking greater humility and
turning oneself over with feminist doctrine. Yet many of the women
I meet in A.A. are strong feminists.
Have you read any Sonia Johnson?

No.

Sonia Johnson is the woman who was thrown out of the Mormon
church because of her stance on women's issues. Anyway, *Wildfire*
is her fourth book. It came out in 1989, and in it she had a wonderful
chapter. She interviewed me just as you are, and after we discussed
things, she entitled a chapter "Twelve Steps into the Fog." She quotes
me a lot there, but she brought out exactly what we're talking about.
And a book that came out just last week is Phyllis Hobe's. She is an
ACOA, a child of an alcoholic, who criticizes that program because

it's totally based on twelve steps. The twelve steps don't deal with the issues of women who are adult children of alcoholics. My theory has always been that these issues are not germane to women who are adult children of alcoholics, or to addicts, or to women alcoholics. We must deal with the problems that are germane to women, period. It has nothing to do with what we're trying to overcome. It has absolutely nothing to do with alcoholism, or little or nothing. That is an illness. It's a disease. And the way that it's treated is to stop drinking. But what you have left is a very upset, confused woman. And she needs a program to deal with problems of her gender, not her alcoholism. Her alcoholism is treated not with pills, not with injections but with cessation of drinking. And then she needs a program that deals with her problems because she is a *woman*, and our problems are almost exactly opposite those of the male. He needs treatment too, but his problems are quite different from ours.

In what way?

Well, for instance, the male alcoholic needs to deal with coming to grips with his feelings. That's why he's so happy to tell his story in A.A. meetings. It keeps him from dealing with his feelings. He's got this nice epic that he can haul out about how he slept with all these broads and so forth and so on.

And women have trouble with that. It keeps them from really delving any deeper into anything of any real consequence in their recovery.

You know, it's interesting—I'm leaving tomorrow morning for Akron, Ohio, for the National Feminist Women's Studies Convention conference, and there will be 4,000 women there. It's about every issue of women and feminism and women's studies. I and three other women submitted abstracts that were accepted, and would you believe that at a feminist conference, three of those four papers are on A.A. Mine is the only one that is not on A.A., so this should be extremely interesting.

Well, from what I gathered you're going to stick to your guns?

Oh, absolutely. I've been at this for sixteen years.

If a woman called you and said "I'm having trouble with A.A." what would you do—send her the literature, talk to her on the phone?

Get her into one of our groups right away. Talk to her. Help her, try to get her to understand what's happening to her. Anybody that contacts us, all they need to do is send a self-addressed stamped envelope and we'll send them the program, our program, how to use it, and where the nearest group is. In the last twenty-four months I've seen more persons beginning to say what we used to whisper, *"A.A. doesn't work for everybody,"* and it's about time we all spoke out. We're not just criticizing them but we're trying to point out that there are other ways to recover, and what we're trying to do has nothing to do with putting A.A. down. We must give A.A. it's greatness, but if it doesn't work, we must not fault ourselves.

July 1990

Kathryn Kennedy King

Thirty-eight, married, and sober since 1987, she is still amazed that it took her so long to recognize her own alcoholism. She was born in San Diego, California, and now lives in Juneau, Alaska. Her father and one of her sisters are also alcoholics. She has finished law school, and is waiting to take the bar exam. She is deeply committed to Women for Sobriety. A determination to stay sober, her positive outlook and levelheadedness, woven around flashes of brilliance, make Kathryn Kennedy King.

I went to high school in the mid-sixties and I became involved in marijuana, LSD, and mescaline. I didn't start doing any heavy drugs until after I got out of high school. I was not a drinker. My parents are alcoholics and I had that example in the home. Also at the time, it was socially unhip to drink alcohol.

My first experience with alcohol was at seventeen and I became very sick. I didn't like the feeling of no control. I didn't know what the word "alcoholic" meant, but as a teenager I felt that a lot of the trauma in my home was alcohol induced. We were middle-class, lived in a nice neighborhood, and my father had a good job. From the outside it looked totally normal, but it was not normal inside. It was very, very dysfunctional, and disrupted by alcohol.

I really didn't start to drink until I was of legal age. I was almost twenty. I started working in bars and my drinking was very controlled.

Alcoholism is one of the major problems in Alaska. We have more alcoholics per capita than any place in the nation. At that time, in the early seventies, we were all partying hardy. I started drinking seriously and having major consequences from my alcohol consumption. I had blackouts. I didn't become violent until later on, but I had incredible mood swings. I became totally uninhibited, and rather promiscuous. I became a different person when I drank. I thought that's what *everybody* did. I had absolutely no information or education on alcoholism. I've realized since I'm recovering that I was an alcoholic from my first experience with alcohol. I ended up kind of trashing my life at a very young age here in Alaska.

I did what is called a geographic. I didn't know that's what I was doing but I went back East to Washington D.C. where my brother was stationed in the army. I stayed there for several years and started working for Amtrak. Through all this I was still involved with all the other drugs. My alcohol consumption did not subside; I just changed locations. I was drinking very heavily in my early twenties, when I was living in Washington. I would sober up and go to work. I never related my problems to alcohol consumption. It was the thing to do at the time, along with all the other drugs. But I remember people saying, "I really think you have a problem with alcohol." I remember thinking, "No problem. I have no more problem with this than I do with any of the other drugs that I'm abusing." My life seemed normal. I was a nice, white, middle-class girl. I had a good job, and an active social life. Without me knowing it, the disease was progressing rapidly.

Then I stopped drinking for a time. I'd been at a party in downtown D.C. and I'd gotten very, very drunk. I decided that I was going to go home. I couldn't find my car and I ended up walking, which was probably a good thing. I don't really remember what happened after that, but I woke up in the pantry of a restaurant. I had gotten cold, broken a window, opened a door and had fallen asleep in the pantry of a restaurant in a blackout. That was pretty scary to me. I *still* didn't know anything about alcoholism. I still didn't know that this was something that was going to progress. I just thought that I should stop drinking, and for a while I did. I was twenty-one years old.

Then I met a guy who was with my brother in the army. We lived together in Washington, D.C. and then in California, and then we came up here. His family is in Fairbanks and mine was in Juneau. We stopped in Juneau to see my family and I didn't want to go any further. It was right in the midst of the construction of the Alaska pipeline. We had heard horror stories about Fairbanks, which we termed the Tijuana of the north. I didn't get along with his father. I decided not to go on to Fairbanks and the relationship ended.

At that point I was still very much caught up in that counter-culture, new age kind of thinking, so I didn't start drinking heavily again for a while. I was heavy into cocaine. But I never quit drinking, I drank beer.

As time went on I got back into the bar business and started drinking and doing cocaine very heavily. I quit doing cocaine on or around my twenty-ninth birthday.

What do you mean by "very heavily"? A quart a day?

No, not that much. Maybe half a quart a day. I really couldn't determine how much because I was working in bars so it wasn't like I had to go out and buy the stuff. I would go to work at six o'clock and I would close the bar. I would drink continuously. Oftentimes, I would take a bottle of whiskey with me when I left and not finish it until the next day or the day after. What happened was that I was so heavily into cocaine—I didn't realize how much I was drinking and was able to drink more without completely losing control or blacking out. This was right before my twenty-ninth birthday and I *still* did not relate any of my problems to alcohol. I didn't think it was a major problem. I just thought it was me; that I was really screwed up and didn't have any direction.

I quit doing cocaine because I was starting to get psychotic. I was paranoid and having feelings of suicide. One thing I should give my family and my background credit for, is that I've never really pushed the envelope. I've never gone over the edge; I've always kind of sensed where the edge was.

You never pushed the envelope?

It's an air force term. How fast and how far you can go. I didn't consciously realize that I was an alcoholic. But subconsciously, there were controls that kept me from going the way so many of my friends went. I never OD'd. I always managed to pull myself up before things got out of hand. I've only had one brush with the criminal justice system and that was for drunk driving. Drinking and driving don't mix, so I quit driving. I always had a sense, some values, intuitive knowledge, or maybe just sheer survival instincts, that kept me from going over the edge with alcohol and drugs. I was always kind of catching myself before things got really bad and either pulling a geographic or changing jobs—whatever it took. While not actually quitting these things, I did slow them down. I was arresting the process for a short period of time.

This all came to a screeching halt on my twenty-ninth birthday. I had a dream which made me realize I just couldn't do this any longer. I decided to leave Juneau and go to college. I didn't have much college under me. I dreamt that I woke up and I walked into one of the local bars and my name was carved on one of the bar stools. I was forty-nine. It was like, whoah. And that's exactly what I said to myself. "I do not want to be doing this in twenty years." It kind of pulled me up by the short hairs.

I got a loan and ended up going to Seattle to college where I was very, very successful. I did four years of college in three years and graduated magna cum laude with a 3.85 grade point average. I got all kinds of awards and accolades. Through all this, I did not quit drinking and drugging. But I prioritized. Being a success in school was very important to me. It felt like it was my last chance to do anything with my life. I put my disease on the back burner.

I was a periodic binger, not so much a daily drinker. I would wait for a three-day weekend. Then I'd go get drunk and do drugs. Since it never interfered with my school life, it was no longer a problem. A couple of my good friends had gone into rehabs and they started telling me about their experiences. This was the beginning of my education on the subject. They started telling me about their treatment and how they felt. I wasn't threatened by it. I was fascinated. I didn't relate it to myself personally or anything. But I listened, and I learned.

I graduated from the university and I was accepted into law school. During my senior year of college I had to have emergency surgery. One of my fallopian tubes became twisted and was cutting off my circulation. I didn't give myself enough time to recover and the operation herniated. The pressure of the hernia started putting pressure on the nerves in my legs. I would be in pain after I walked or stood up or did anything for very long. I became more sedentary and I started gaining weight.

I was in law school, which was not like undergrad at all. It was very hard. It wasn't even so much that it was so hard; it wasn't nurturing. I had come from a very, very nurturing university environment to a very harsh and competitive environment. It was really kind of frightening and I discovered, to my surprise, that I was still an idealist. I really had trouble with law school. My ambition was to be a yuppie, but it wasn't working. Because of this idealism, there were a lot of emotional and philosophical conflicts in law school.

My disease was progressing. I wasn't thinking straight. The nerve damage was keeping me from being as active as I had once been and I was putting on weight, which was making the nerve damage worse. I would drink for the pain. By Christmas of '87, I was drinking about a quart a day. Doing simple tasks like loading the dishwasher would cause me a lot of pain. I would wake up in the morning and put Grand Marnier in my coffee and that's how I would drink. Grand Marnier in my coffee all day until early afternoon, then I would start drinking vodka and sodas until evening, when I would start drinking Bombay on the rocks.

I met my fiance the summer before my last year as an undergraduate. It was right after they had voted down the move to switch the Alaska capital from Juneau to Anchorage. So Juneau was really partying and this went on for a couple of years. Business boomed and everybody had a lot of money. Dan and I partied real heavy together. He loved me, loved me, loved me. He isn't an alcoholic and he doesn't come from alcoholic parents. I'd never met anybody like that. He didn't really have any understanding of the disease.

He was an incredibly successful enabler. From the very beginning I had drunken tantrums. But he would just kind of overlook that because I was so wonderful when I was sober. Of course we had problems—all the problems people have in relationships when one person is alcoholic and the other person loves them very much and is unwilling to let them go. We would go out and spend just fortunes on dinner and drinks. He'd buy all my girlfriends drinks. I would get plowed and I would be just horrible to him. This went on for half of our relationship.

The day after Christmas in 1987 we had a Christmas party. Everything just went swimmingly. I was very uptight about this party but it went very well. Our family and Dan's boss and all our friends came. I drank a quart of Bombay by myself that night. Everything went fine until everybody left. I blacked out and to this day I don't know exactly what set me off. Over the last three years I've reconstructed a lot of it. I went into an insane rage: I broke dishes, I knocked the television over, I pulled a knife on Dan. I broke glass. I trashed the entire house. The only thing I remember is that the police were there. My sister had come to the party with a friend of ours so instead of arresting me, the police let me go with my sister and her friend. Dan called the police, not because he was afraid of me, but because he was afraid of himself and of what he would do to me. I think I even took a bottle of gin with me. Of course I was so indignant. How could he possibly do this, the asshole, I don't need him and blah, blah, blah and so forth.

I went over to a friend's and slept it off. But I didn't sleep very long. I woke up. I was still pretty intoxicated but I thought I was sober. I called a cab and I went back home. I was still real indignant. "I don't need this shit." As I was packing up my stuff I realized that he was *helping* me. After everything was packed up, I passed out. He woke me up at about six and said, "It's getting dark, I think you should call your father to come get you." I said, "I'm not going anywhere." He said, "Yes, you are. I love you, but it's gotten to where being with you is so much more painful than not. I can't go on like this." I knew. The pain. My denial shattered in that very second. I looked at him and I started to say, "Well, I can't promise you anything. . . . " But then I realized I had to promise him because he was serious. This was it. I looked at his face and I saw the pain and bewilderment, the suffering, and I just broke. When I think about it, I always say the "shattering of my denial" because I see my denial as a glass or Lucite compartment I lived in. I see my denial as shattered pieces of glass all around me. It could have been all the broken glass in the apartment, I don't know. But that's always been the symbol for me of what happened. I realized in the depths of my soul that I was an alcoholic and that alcohol was ruining my life. That was my first realization that that was an absolute fact. Dan let me stay.

And you decided to do something?

Well, I didn't really know exactly what to do. I cried and I told him how sorry I was and that I would get help and I said, "I promise that this will never, ever happen again." And he believed me. And it never, ever has happened again. I think it's *because* he believed me.

The next day I asked my sister to come over. My sister is nine years younger than I am. We're very, very close. She's my best friend and I'm her best friend. I told her everything—about breaking into that place and a lot of the ugly little stories that I was so ashamed of. It seemed like a real natural thing to do; just pull out the ugliness and lay it out. I mean, this was really a do-it-yourself attitude for a recovery program. It just seemed like I needed to tell somebody how totally disgusting I had been under the influence of alcohol. I didn't want to do that to Dan because it just wasn't fair. My sister loves me, loves me, loves me. And it was like I was vomiting years and years of bile—about the people I had ended up sleeping with and ripping off. I told her all the really disgusting things that I'd done while drinking.

And you were still in law school?

Yes, I was still in law school. That's the amazing thing about this. I've come to the conclusion that I'm either very, very stupid or very, very smart. I don't know which one it is yet. I couldn't give up. Part of the breakthrough in the experience that I had, when my denial broke down, was that I saw the rest of my life as a drain. I hated law school. I hated myself. I hated everything. I'd alienated myself from just about everyone. My family was fed up with me. Dan was the only really good thing left in my life. If I lost him, I would not have remained in law school. It would have been a downward spiral. I also felt that I was throwing myself off a cliff and that he, at great personal risk, stood in my way. Our relationship has balanced out, eased out, but at that time he was in so much danger. I loved him so much and I knew he loved me. But he was cold serious when he said those things to me . . . there was no doubt about it. That was the end and I knew it.

I didn't go to A.A. right away. I started thinking about the things that two of my friends, who had been recovering while I was in college, had told me. I went to the library and got some books. I read and started talking to people. I realized that I knew a lot of people who had stopped drinking. I was depressed for days, I was so disgusted with myself. Dan made me go to the grocery store on

New Year's Eve. He said it would be good for me. My first en-
counter, I guess, with working on my feelings about being sober
was the next day, New Year's Day in 1988. We had been invited to
a football party and I did not want to go. There was going to be
alcohol. The friends that we had partied with were going to be there.
I magnanimously said to Dan, "You go ahead and go." But I was
just crushed when he did. I was really upset. It hurt my feelings and
that's when it dawned on me, right then and there. I wanted to have
a drink, I said, "Wow, there's a real connection between your hurt
feelings and your need to drink." I ran a hot bath and got in the
bathtub and cried. I let my feelings be heard. I realized at that point
that the way to stay sober was to acknowledge the feelings that made
me want to drink. Nothing was more important to me than staying
sober. And so I embarked on my do-it-yourself recovery program.

And so you never did go to A.A.?

Not really. I went to a couple of meetings. I bought the Big Book
and read the stories. I paid attention to the steps and learned a lot. I
have always used a lot of A.A. things because they felt right and it
really worked for me. There's good stuff that I pass on to other
people about A.A. It's great stuff, but I had problems with it from
the very beginning. It reminded me of fundamental religion. I was
really successfully doing it at home; a do-it-yourself recovery program. I called it the "small triumph" theory of recovery. I had a lot
of support—my husband, my sister, my father, my mom. It was
just like everything was kind of laid out for me. It was very surrealistic in that when I did learn more of the principles of A.A., I
realized how good and right on it was. I experienced it completely.
It wasn't like I had to force it. It was a blinding revelation of who I
was and what alcohol had done to me, and the fact that I wasn't that
under-the-influence person. I was somebody completely different
from that drunken, angry, tough person I thought I was. I didn't
have to learn that slowly, painfully. It just happened. I was able to
make the distinction even before I read anything. I knew what needed
to be done, from conversations with my friends that had been
through rehabs and from my own instincts. I was so motivated to
stay sober. I really loved this man and I saw the breakdown of my
denial as a miracle. It was so clear to me what my problem was and

what I had to do. I don't think everybody is fortunate enough to have such a devastating realization.

I was real frightened of A.A. I can't deny that. I still don't know why. I have had emotional relapses and I've had one drinking experience in the three years I've been sober. That was a year ago. I flunked the bar the first time and my husband—we were married after I graduated from college—had given me a ticket to see the Rolling Stones in Vancouver for their '89 tour. He thought that it would be a nice consolation prize for me. It was symbolically kind of the bookend of my teenage years. The last time I had seen the Stones was in 1969 and so I figured I had gone through this incredible twenty-year teen-age since then.

How do you feel about that, relapsing?

Well, I had a real good time but I was with strangers, and was away from my home.

Was it because you failed the bar?

No, I can't say that. I think that was part of it. Last year was a very, very emotional, traumatic time for me. A lot of things come into play here. It wasn't just failing the bar, although that was a catalytic event. My mother died in 1988 when I'd been sober four months. She died rather suddenly, and my father, who had been sober for five years prior to my mother's death, started drinking very, very heavily again. My sister, who had stopped drinking when I had, started drinking again. My brother in Anchorage and my sister in California started going through very messy divorces and custody battles and their children, whom I loved dearly, were being yanked. I was the only sober, functioning member of my family. And, of course, being a child of alcoholics, I had assumed that responsible role of fixer. I had to make everybody better. And because I was sober and married to this wonderful man, and my life was so rosy, I felt I should be able to fix everyone else's life. Well, I came to discover, about a year and a half later, that I couldn't fix anybody.

I lost touch with my own recovery program. I had started smoking pot again. I was not drinking alcohol and I was half-heartedly work-

ing the steps and going to meetings, but everything was a real struggle. It was almost as if I totally postponed my own grieving because
I was so busy caretaking everybody else in my family. So when I
got my bar results and Dan sent me off to Vancouver to have this
wonderful party with the Rolling Stones, it all came crashing down
on me. The disease reared its ugly head. It said, "You can do this,
you're going to be different this time." But I wasn't any different.
I wasn't violent or promiscuous, but I was an asshole. I was really
lucky because there weren't any bad, major consequences to my
doing this. Nothing had changed. To think that I could ever drink
socially was a crock.

I forgave myself for it completely because it was so funny actually.
Now that I'm involved with Women for Sobriety and I'm doing
some amateur counseling, I have a lot more empathy because I *have*
relapsed. It was only one day, one time. I feel very fortunate for that
because I just knew, "No, you didn't sleep with anyone. No, you
didn't lose anything. You didn't beat anybody up. You even had a
good time. But you can't drink, and you'll never be able to drink."

Is that when you decided to join Women for Sobriety?

No. I didn't know about Women for Sobriety. I came back and I
tried to go to A.A. meetings. God, talk about the tortures of the
damned. This is rather a small community and so Alcoholics Anonymous isn't anonymous. I mean, all the alcoholics know each other
real well and because I had such trouble going to meetings I would
maybe go once a month. I knew the schedule by memory and I could
tell everyone else when a meeting was, but I never showed up. I felt
really guilty. When I did show up, I would get this feeling that
everyone thought I had been sitting in a bar someplace, that I wasn't
really sober all this time. It became a real problem for me.

After Christmas I went into private counseling to deal with things.
My father, as it turns out, at Christmas time, bottomed out completely and we had to admit him to the hospital to be detoxed. My
sister bottomed out. I bottomed out. It was a real mess. I never drank
again, but I was still not recovering. It was a real bad time and I was
very, very caught up in the family disease.

I was so angry at my father. In my opinion, he was besmirching
the memory of my mother. He wasn't drinking because she died,

he was using her death as an excuse to drink. My relationship with my father was nil. I couldn't even talk to him, I was so angry. I was getting it coming and going. I had my own guilt for not doing anything about the situation and then my sister would lay a bunch of guilt on me because I wasn't helping her. We decided when we put Dad in the hospital that no matter what he did, we both needed help. We could not go on like this. We both sought private counseling. I worked on my feelings about A.A. and my problems with my father. . . .

What do you think your feelings about A.A. were?

I had real negative feelings about it. I'm not angry with it any more. You know, you read the Big Book and you read the literature and there's that promise of fellowship. And you see the old movies . . . but I never, ever experienced that. Never once experienced that feeling of welcome, of non-judgmentalness. I never felt fellowship, and I went to quite a few different meetings. I felt kind of betrayed by that. I felt that it was very competitive. "Who's the better alcoholic?" I certainly was not a very good alcoholic because I wasn't doing ninety meetings in ninety days. I wasn't making coffee and I only showed up once a month. I was upset with that. They said, "We're going to go to your house and we're going to clear out your vanilla extract and your cough medicine." And I said, "Well, if you're going to do that, why don't you start with the liquor closet? My husband is not an alcoholic and there has always been alcohol in my house. It's not a problem with me. And I'm sorry, I'm not going to throw away my vanilla extract because I haven't found myself chug-a-lugging it yet." Just things like that.

I have a real aversion to fanaticism, either religious or political faddiness. I have an aversion to it; I find it a dangerous thing instinctively. And that's what I felt from A.A. *This is the only way and if you don't do it this way, follow these rules and believe these tenets, you're going to hell.*

You're not going to stay sober is what they say, and I found that not to be true.

I didn't start to recover in A.A, I started to recover within myself, with things I discovered that instinctively worked for me. Total honesty with yourself is the paramount key, as painful as that may be. That's the hardest part, but that is the key to recovery.

Something else that has really helped me a great deal is recovering from marijuana abuse. I discovered after I quit drinking that marijuana was my primary drug of choice. I can really understand what some alcoholics go through because of my struggle with pot. I joined Women for Sobriety when I really needed to work on my marijuana use.

Denise, the moderator for Women for Sobriety, was running public service announcements and I had read about Women for Sobriety years earlier in a Dear Abby column. My counselor had been telling me I really needed some group activity. I kept saying, "I hate A.A. You can't make me go to A.A." I called Denise and I didn't let myself hesitate. She came over that very day, and I was so attracted to her. She's very courageous, up and very confident. And I thought, "Wow, I want what this person has and I want to be a part of this and I want to be her friend." So I have committed myself wholeheartedly to Women for Sobriety. One of the things about Women for Sobriety is that it is so very much like what I did for myself before I knew about it, when I just couldn't gel with A.A. but was recovering through my own self-evaluation, through giving myself many, many strokes. Whatever the incident was that made me want to drink, I would think, "Why do I want to drink?" And I would work through that and then I wouldn't drink. Then I would call someone who supported me and they would be very proud of me and I would be very proud of myself. That was how I recovered. I had people who really, really supported my recovery process.

Everyone needs Women for Sobriety. And it certainly doesn't have to exclude A.A. There isn't a woman alive, regardless of her status with substance problems, who can't get this program to work for her. It is a recovery program. It is a self-esteem building program, and it works.

November 1990

Lynn

Lynn is twenty-nine years old. The daughter of a bar owner in Alabama, she is married to Keith, twenty-eight, also a recovering alcoholic. Keith is in the military, and their life together has been a series of moves. Five feet five and slender, she combines a homecoming queen's beauty with short blonde curly hair and vivid features. Her smoker's cough mingles with her laugh. I caught her in Chicopee, Massachusetts, between moves. She and Keith had just returned from a five-year tour of duty in West Germany. A devoted member of Alcoholics Anonymous, Lynn bubbles over with excitement and talks nonstop. Her personality radiates warmth. She is so excited about being sober that she can't wait to tell her story. When she was drinking, she says, her behavior was violent, insolent, and angry. I sense that Lynn often says to herself, "How did I get stuck with this disease?" Her eyes occasionally well up with tears, but she always manages to hold back. "I can't cry," she says. "It's one of my biggest problems." She has been sober since 1986. Ironically, she has become the popular, outgoing person she was trying to be when she started to drink. Lynn attends A.A. meetings and Adult Children of Alcoholics (ACOA) meetings. She reads whatever she can find about alcoholism.

I'll tell you a little bit of my family history. My mother was a product of all of her mother's unresolved coping mechanisms. Her mother was abusive. And my mother carried that on down through the family. She joined the Women's Army Corps. She met my father there and he drank alcoholically. What I consider alcoholically. When they met, they met in clubs. They hung out in bars. I took a brief family history just last week back home in Keene, New Hampshire, where I was raised. I talked to uncles and aunts and cousins—it's all there . . . multi-generational alcoholism. There's a lot of us in the family. It's considered normal. And I see where kids my age, or younger, consider drinking normal.

I was raised where Grammie going out crocked at two o'clock in the morning, and beating up the bushes because the azaleas wouldn't bloom, was normal. There was a shame about it that I hid inside, wondering if there was something wrong here. It was real confusing. I didn't trust my feelings because I said, "Grammie's fine. She's just having a good time."

When did you start drinking?

When I was thirteen, at a junior high dance. I always felt like a round peg trying to fit into a square hole. Always. That phrase just fit me. I wasn't shy. I was a permanent victim. I was picked on in school, nobody liked me. I had one friend. I was picked last for softball. Nobody wanted to be on the other end of the jump rope. I felt very lonely. And that song, I can't think of the name of it, a lady sings it; at seventeen, sitting around waiting for the phone to ring.

I never went to a prom. Drinking was the hidden key. That was it. That was the answer. That was what was missing—that feeling of, "I'm okay," just settled over me when I drank. It felt warm. I was standing outside a junior high dance. A little bottle was going around. Of course I was always alone, and so I said, "Shoot. This is my way in, I'll be a big guy," and stepped up and drank with the girls. That was it. I was the best dancer, I was the most popular person there. All my inhibitions left. I had that boost of self-confidence. I could go and do it all. The one friend I always had was in it with me.

How did your drinking progress?

My father had a bar in Alabama, so it was real easy to drink. One night I was alone, outside, and I was drinking. A car drove up and

I got into the car with someone I didn't know and I put myself in a real unsafe position and I got raped. I didn't tell anyone about the rape because I was drinking. I didn't think about the rape. I thought about it in terms of my drinking—I'd get killed for drinking. This is what I told myself. I'd done so many things wrong for so long.

My mother and father got divorced when I was four. One year we lived with my mother in New Hampshire, the next with my father in Alabama. The army life is perfect for me. I was raised for the army life. We moved so often. At my father's bar, in Alabama, I would sneak drinks in the back. I was the cook and dishwasher— a typical compulsive worker. You never knew when you might slip up and blow it. But I would be covered because I was such a good worker. I drank a lot then, but denied it because "everyone else in here does it."

I was very codependent at the time. I was worried about my dad, so if anything was said to me about my drinking I would compare it to my father or brothers, and then it was normal. Or I was the one with the least of the problems. I was always the hero. The good kid. The one who didn't get in trouble and did the best. Seems like there was only room in my dad's heart for two of us; there were three of us. One always had to be the scapegoat. That's real normal in ACOA families too. I didn't know that then. If you weren't one of the good ones in there you were the scapegoat. I was a scapegoat for my mom. I wasn't willing to be one for my dad.

At seventeen I drank more. In our home it was okay to have a beer around Dad. Dad would bring home a six-pack. "Hey, can I have one?" "Sure, go ahead." There was no problem with that. So for me, it was like popping a Coke. It was never questioned.

Where did you drink?

Off with friends or alone.

Were you a social drinker?

Yeah, yeah. I was an alcoholic drinker, but I considered it social drinking. Stuff you bragged about on Tuesday at school. All of us were drinking, so I didn't really stand out. We moved again to another part of Alabama. My father's drinking had progressed to the violent drunk. He would come home at two or three in the morning, drunk, and get everybody in the house out of bed. We'd go into the living room and listen to him preach about what worthless kids we were. He'd say, "Cook something." "There's nothing in the refrigerator to cook. What do you want me to cook?" "There's beans in the cabinet." "Well, beans take ten hours." But I stood there and stirred at the stove anyway. He was in a fog and didn't know what I was cooking anyway.

Dad got real violent one night with my little brother. Beat the tar out of him. I mean all over the living room, and I was terrified. I thought, "Oh, no. This is it." He had done things before but he had never touched any one of us. When it got to bodies being thrown around, I got terrified.

I felt like the wife. I had taken the wife role. He was single and it was us three kids. I did the laundry, the cooking, that sort of thing. I didn't have the guts to confront him then. I was seventeen and not allowed to date. It was two weeks before my eighteenth birthday and it was like I was his wife. I didn't know this was abnormal. I slept with my father until I was seventeen. I didn't have sex with him. (Whispers.) I didn't know this wasn't normal until I saw a counselor, and said, "I slept with my dad." And he said, "That's not normal." "It's *not?* I didn't know." And he said, "Did you have sex with him?" "No." "You're lucky because that's a very incestuous relationship. That's dangerous." I felt like my father's wife instead of his girlfriend—uh oh, Freudian slip—daughter.

The next morning I wrote a note to my dad. I went to a friend's house and called my mom long distance. I said, "Send tickets." Tickets were in the mail the next day. We left. That was it. It was never discussed. I felt elated to be getting out of that situation. Finally, something new. It will be different. (Laughs.) The alcoholic's geographical cure.

Did you feel that you were abandoning your father?

Yes. I knew something was wrong. I felt like, "Who's going to take care of him now?"

What happened when you got to your mom's?

I went to a counselor within a week. I just felt insane. Insane. That's the only word I can think of. Just totally out of control of my life. I went to a counselor and he said, "Did it ever occur to you that your father might be an alcoholic?" And I said, (whispers) "Jesus Christ, don't say that." Now my father's twelve hundred miles away. This is the control I thought he had. "If he hears you, you're going to be dead. He's gonna kick my butt. He's gonna take me back there. Don't even think it." He still has control. The counselor said, "I want you to come back in two days. We need to talk." I went back one more time. He told me that I'm beautiful. I started crying. He said I was special. I said, "Please, don't say that." It's what I believed way way way way down, under all this crap. There was so much garbage and it felt safe to have all the garbage covering it up. It was unsafe, and not okay to feel good about myself. He said not to get into any relationships right now. "You're too vulnerable. You just left a real chaotic home. It would be normal for you to find a new relationship, and it would be worse." I said, "Oh, be serious." I wasn't ready to hear what he was saying. He said, "Let's bring your mom and your brother in. If you want to get better, it would be a good idea if you were all in here getting better together."

So we all went in together and sat down and I was a clown. I did everything I could to sabotage that. Everything—I wanted it so bad, but I was terrified.

You wanted to get healthy, but it frightened you?

Right. Because there is a certain sense of security in the familiar. Exactly. Unpredictability at that time would have terrified me. All I knew was the sick kind of unpredictability.

But you were still drinking?

Yeah, I was still drinking. Just whatever I could get. I think at this point I was acting out of codependence more than anything else. I was a shadow drinker. As long as there was someone else out front being the focus of attention, then I could do whatever I wanted and nobody would really pay that much attention to me.

Just before I left my dad, he said, "I am going to predict your future for you. Within six months you are going to be out of school. You're going to be pregnant. You're going to be married, and you're going to be miserable." That shows me the insidiousness, the insanity of this disease. Because no father wants that for his daughter, but the insanity of the disease makes garbage like that come out of it. It's better for me to be angry at the disease than angry at my father. I've got to get past the anger. There's a lot I want to talk to him about—separating the little girl from the daddy. I want us to be friends. I want to get rid of some of the garbage and get on.

I got married, had my two children, and became a serious over-eater. I weighed 209 pounds. I was obese. I married an alcoholic. He was very mild, addicted to TV. I don't really remember myself drinking much at all. The last good drunk I remember was the night I got married. I had a big bash. Then after that I don't remember being drunk until two years later. I was twenty-one. The man I married, he turned out to be a transvestite. I was relieved. It was somebody else's problem for a change. He went to Korea. I knew the marriage was over. There was no salvaging it. I just knew. I couldn't ask him to change. Oddly enough, I couldn't live with it either so I made the choice. I got out.

Do you think his drinking made it easier for you not to drink?

It could have. I started drinking right after that, so that makes sense.

Did you stop eating when you started drinking again?

Yes. My mom always called me roly-poly, chubby. I always had this vision that I was fat, fat, fat. I look back at the pictures and I wasn't fat, I was cute.

I moved back to Fort Campbell, Kentucky. I started drinking heavy. I said, "Ma, take the kids. He's not giving me child support. Can you take the kids until I get a job?" Reality was that I was drinking so much that I couldn't control my children, my home life,

and a working life. There was just no way. The drinking was interfering. I thought it was the children and the lack of financial
support. I was drinking to the point where I couldn't get up in the
morning. With little babies you have to get up. You're supposed to
get up and feed them and make sure they have a bath. I just thought,
"They'll take care of themselves; I have to take care of myself." I
was losing it. So I took the kids to New Hampshire and I went back
to Fort Campbell. I felt horrible. I felt at least they'll be able to eat;
someone would take care of them, they'd have a semi-secure home.
I didn't think I was personally capable. I know better now. I was
capable. I chose to drink.

I gave up the kids to my mom in January. I met Keith. I got my
first DWI. Talk about embarrassing. I got a $3,000 dollar fine, a
$250 lawyer fee, an $80 court cost, and 48 hours in jail plus a year's
suspension on my driver's license. I'm in this grey room with a
woman I knew was a junkie and these two obese women. I thought
to myself, "This isn't right. I don't belong in here. This is a mistake."
We were all suffering from the same sort of disease in one way or
another and we're all in jail. It was just horrible. I knew all the cops
and they arrested me anyway. They let me down. I tried joking my
way out of it; nothing worked. Two days in jail seemed like two
years. I know what they mean by the clank of the door. They gave
you a rolled-up mattress. It was horrible.

I had met Keith and he was my only hope of getting out of there.
"Someday when I get out of here . . ." I said, "When I get out of
here, he's my answer. I was looking for a Sir Galahad, a knight in
shining armor, someone to rescue me from this horrible world that
was doing terrible things to me. My life was out of control. He was
there and he's got a rescue complex. When I got out I was still
drinking.

I changed jobs right after I got out. I found there was more money
in dancing with a bathing suit on than there was in waitressing. But
I had to be crocked to get up there. At first I looked at that as an
excuse to get drunk. God, the shame when I think about what I must
have looked like up there drunk. I made lots of money but it went
to drinking.

We got a trailer and I asked my mom to send the kids back. Keith
and I were living together. He was in the army and I was dancing.
I couldn't get up in the morning with my kids. Keith was the hero.
He was there, but he had to go to work. He would wake me up. I

was hung over every single day. I lost concept of time. Social welfare was called in because my children weren't being taken care of.

We moved to Georgia for the army, to Germany for the army. It started all over again. The drinking, the fights, the violence. We had both gotten violent. When we came home on leave before we went to Germany, he whacked his toe off with the lawnmower. He thought his army career was over, and that to him was everything. He was gone all the time and I was back into codependence.

What made you decide you wanted to quit drinking?

We got to Germany and the violence continued between us. There were street brawls and bar fights. It never got to the point of physical violence between us until one night he was drinking and I was not— one of us had to be in semi-control. He beat the shit out of me. That night the fighting continued and continued until one o'clock in the morning. He just snapped, that was it. All of a sudden he lost control, blacked out, and beat the shit out of me. When the soldiers picked me up, they took me to their barracks. It's mandatory that you call the Military Police. It was automatically reported. That's what saved me. Most abused spouses say, "Oh well, I really don't want to"— they told me I would be threatened with perjury if I took my statement back, so there was no way out of it. I went to the police station. *"He's such a nice guy. You don't know."*

He went to what was called the Rehabilitation Treatment Facility (RTF—a program based on A.A.) for six weeks. He had weekend passes and came home and he was telling me that this is really neat stuff. I'm thinking, "Uh oh," little red lights were flashing. "I'm next." I knew I had to change or get out of the situation. It's just the way it's always been. I had always chosen to get out of the situation. But this was my life. He was the only stability I had. I couldn't leave him being as codependent as I was, it didn't matter.

At RTF, they made the spouse go for the final two weeks of the six-week in-house program. That's when I started opening my eyes. And I signed myself up at the end of that six weeks to go back for my own six weeks. I would be the recovering alcoholic and he would come for my last two weeks. That was three years ago, September.

What was that like?

It was tough love. They would hug me and I would freeze. I never knew what to expect. I still quote what I heard there. Everything I heard there is still right here (points to her head). You go in and have a group. There's no bullshit allowed. It is straight up, they called you on it. Every other word out of your mouth—"that's bullshit." I would get so frustrated. "What do you want me to say?" And they would say, "We want to hear the honest truth." "What is the truth?" "I don't know what the truth is." And I was honest. I didn't know what the truth was. So I hated it. The first three weeks I kicked my feet. "Fine, I'll just come in here and sit." But if you don't open your mouth, and you're not recovering, there's ten thousand *other* people out there that need this seat, so we're just going to kick you out. They were tough. They said that if you don't open your mouth, you're out of here. "No, goddammit, I'm not getting thrown out of here." I started crying. I was hysterical. "There's no way. I want this disease to leave me. I know I am powerless. I can't handle it anymore. My life is unmanageable. I feel insane. Everything is going crazy and I want to talk about it." "Oh, finally some honesty is coming out." (Laughs.) Oh, that place, I hated it. Then things got better and I didn't want to leave at the end of my six weeks.

What was the first year of sobriety like?

It was insane. Everything. There were issues everywhere. My sponsor was tough. She had five years in the program. She said, "You are not going to deal with your marriage this year. You're not dealing with anything." So, I dealt with sobriety. That was enough. Learning how to live sober was enough. I never had the craving to drink. I craved the good times, the dancing, the lights, the music, but I didn't crave the actual physical drink because I hated the taste of it always. Smelling it on someone's breath turned my stomach. I kept looking for chaos and crisis and it wasn't there. It was so hard not to stir shit up when shit felt normal.

Did you ever feel like you might start drinking again?

No. I knew. It didn't matter what happened. I went to five meetings a week in Germany. I had to my first year. I was travelling thirty-five miles in either direction to get there. It was tough.

How do you feel about being a woman in recovery?

Alienated sometimes. It's different being a woman. Yes, I have sexual issues. It's tough to get in a room and talk about hormone problems, or living with a male alcoholic. I think there's so many prejudices. Why does an alcoholic have so many? It would be tough for me to go in there and believe that these people have a totally open mind about what I'm going to say. I was promiscuous. I was giving away huge chunks of myself. Trying to deal with these issues in an all-male group is tough. So I don't. I deal with them through my sponsor.

What about the heredity factor, in terms of your children?

We came out of the RTF and sat down at the table with the kids and said, "Mommy and daddy have a disease we're dealing with called alcoholism and addiction." And they said, "We know that when you drink you get crazy and do stupid things." They go to Al-Atot, for children with alcoholic parents. There is nothing that can't be discussed. Bless their hearts. I also believe that my children will be a product of all my unresolved issues.

Do you think you'll ever drink again?

We're going through all kinds of shit now and I haven't had a drink yet. The thing I have to worry about is those ordinary Tuesdays. I thrive on crisis and chaos. Tuesdays don't have a feeling to them. It's not a Monday or a Friday. It's an ordinary Tuesday. I think I have another drunk in me. I'm not sure I have another getting sober in me. I can't imagine having a belly full of whiskey and a head full of A.A. It's a slow death. The guilt I would feel, the shame, the feeling of letting myself down.

Is there anything else you want to say?

Yes. You can't ride a fence. Either you're an alcoholic or not. Everybody has to make that choice. I'm the only person that can make the decision for myself. I'm it. I have to do it whether I like it or not. I don't have to like it but I do have to do it.

December 1989

Part Six

Nice Girls Don't Drink

I know you drink on the quiet and I know
how much you drink. . . . I've been intending
to tell you to stop your elaborate pretenses
and drink openly if you want to. Do you think
I give a damn if you like your brandy?

> —Rhett Butler talking to Scarlett
> O'Hara,
> *Gone with the Wind*

Hannah

Twenty-seven years old, she is recovering from bulimia as well as alcoholism. The young woman who said, "I was sweet Hannah, nobody suspected me," has become, in sobriety, the sweet woman she claims to have been falsely portraying. She told her story as if in one long breath: exhaling ten years of eating and throwing up, drinking and throwing up; then drinking and eating to forget. She works for an advertising agency in Boston. Five feet two, she weighs one hundred and eighteen pounds. She comes from a wealthy family and is the youngest of seven. She met her fiance in Alcoholics Anonymous. She has been sober since 1987.

My alcoholism really started with food. It may sound odd, but a lot of women in A.A. have food addictions and eating disorders. As an early teenager I began controlling the food in my life. I began controlling how much I ate, when I ate, how many calories, how much exercise I'd have to do to burn *off* those calories.

I proceeded with that for a couple of years. Dieting and exercising. I was fifteen when I took my first drink. I'll never forget it, it was a lot of fun. I had a great time. I had started drinking around seven in the evening, and by ten I was drunk, and happy; just laughing and playing and joking. That evening I almost ended up in bed with some man I didn't even know. I'd never had sex before and I didn't know what I was doing. And I was saved from that situation by some friends. When I woke up the next day I felt horrible. I was very sick. I also felt really bad about the situation I'd gotten myself into. But a part of me was thrilled by that. Living on the edge. It was my first taste of doing something really bad.

I remember feeling lonely in my teenage years, lonely and afraid of life. As a family we moved quite a few times. I ended up going to four different high schools, which made me feel very alone. I was constantly making friends, then making new ones. Consequently I became very good at making friends. I had to. It was a question of survival. I needed to fit in every time we moved. I began noticing that I had a very hard time saying no to people. I always wanted to make people happy; I always wanted to make them like me. And I was very successful at it. Nobody really knew me very well, and when I think back, I didn't know myself. I was a chameleon, I changed colors. I changed my personality and attitudes to fit in wherever I needed to.

The thing I never told anybody was that I felt very afraid and inadequate. Things started getting bad for me when I graduated from high school. I started bingeing and vomiting and being a bulimic. My parents fully expected me to go on to college. I didn't want to. But I went ahead and applied to schools. I got accepted to a number of schools and I didn't want to go to any of them. I wanted to wait a year. My parents asked me if I had anything better in mind to do and I said, "No." They said, "Well, why don't you just try it?" So I went off to college.

How did it start, the throwing up?

One day I ate an enormous amount of sweets. And I decided that the best way to get rid of it, because I didn't want to get fat, was to throw it up. That was something I wish I had never done. If I had known what was in store for me . . . I think I would have killed myself right then and there. I often drank because when I ate large amounts of food and then went and threw up, my throat would hurt. So I'd take a glass of wine or something to numb my throat and sort of numb my stomach out. It would make me feel kind of relaxed. It would help me forget a little bit about what I had just done.

In college I started meeting a lot of men who wanted to go out and drink and go to parties. I really wasn't interested in doing very much school work, so I didn't. I thought that I would make it at

college without having to *do* anything. I was in such a fog. I think
I was in such denial about what was happening that it didn't even
occur to me that if I wasn't doing the work, I would probably flunk
out.

*What do you think made you want to eat like that? Can you
remember?*

I've thought about that a lot. I think that I was stuffing a lot of
feelings. I was really afraid of becoming—I know it may sound silly,
but I was really afraid of becoming a woman. Becoming someone
that people would think of as an adult. I didn't want to grow up. I
didn't want to be having boyfriends. I didn't want to have sex. I
was afraid of leaving home. I don't think there was any one thing.
It's just that there was a lot of anxiety in me. I'd had years of trying
to keep my weight down to look thin and pretty.

Did you plan binges?

Oh yes. I was taking anywhere from forty to sixty dollars out of
the bank and going and buying just tons of food. I'd bring it back
and either prepare it or, not wanting to wait until it got prepared,
I'd just eat it. I've thought a lot about why. What were the emotions
that were going on? I think I just hated myself. I'm not even sure
why. I hated myself and eating was such a pleasure. I loved the taste
of it. I was angry that I couldn't eat as much as I wanted to because
I would get fat. This just seemed like a perfect way.

I flunked out of school. It only took three months to flunk out. I
ended up coming home, and started bingeing and drinking more
than ever. I was still in the stage where food was my main addiction.
I started going out and buying food, lots of food, to binge on. I was
lying to friends and family about what I was doing and why I couldn't
go out. I was stealing money from my family or my friends. I just
didn't care. I didn't care how much time I wasted, how much money
I wasted, or what this was going to do to me. It was just an all-out
obsession. I thought about food constantly. All day long. When could
I have my next binge? When could I throw it up? Where was I going
to throw it up? And it just continued.

I got myself back in college the following year and binged my way through an entire year at another school. At that school, I began drinking a lot more. On the weekends I would go out with girlfriends. After bingeing all day Saturday, I'd go out and drink and smoke cigarettes until three in the morning, then I'd come home in the middle of the night and throw up all the alcohol and whatever food I had left in me. I'd get up Sunday and I'd do it all over again. I'd try to do a little bit of work so I could stay enrolled. It went on for months and months. I stopped doing everything else. I had done some skiing and running. Slowly I dropped all extracurricular activities. Just living to binge and drink.

What were you eating?

Mostly sweets, cakes and cookies. But I would binge on anything, whatever was around. I remember a couple of times cooking whole turkeys and sometimes eating them half raw because I didn't want to wait until they were cooked. I would buy bottles of sweet liqueurs and sip them slowly while I ate and threw up. Alcohol was still not the main addiction, and I don't know if I'll ever be sure if it became the main one. All I know is that alcohol and my bingeing were tied so closely together that I could not recover from one without dropping both of them.

By this time I was having sex with just about anybody that would have it. I had some discretion, some taste, but for the most part I was having sex with a lot of people. I think an important part of my story is that I didn't know how to say no to anything. If there was something I didn't want to do, I would lie my way out of it. I wouldn't say no. And I think one of the biggest gifts I've been given in sobriety is the ability to say, "No. No thank you. I don't want to do that." It took me years to know that that was all right.

I left the next college because I decided I hated it and I wanted to be somewhere else. I thought things would be better somewhere else. I clearly remember the day that I left school. I was on my way, moving to another city and I binged the entire way. I got out and I found a public bathroom and I started throwing up. That night, with my new roommates, I went out and got wasted. That was pretty much the way things went for months and months.

When you eat like that and you throw up, does it really stop you from gaining weight?

Well, it did for a couple of years. When I was in my third year of bingeing I wasn't able to throw up all of the food. It exhausted me to keep trying to throw up everything that I'd eaten, so I began to gain weight. Occasionally I used laxatives. A couple of times I drank some stuff that is sort of a mild poison so that I could throw up even more. When I noticed I was gaining weight I resorted to using Ipecac. It wouldn't kill you but it made you so sick that it would make you throw up. It cost a dollar a bottle at the drug store. Today, when I think of the taste, oh, it makes me ill. It just makes my mouth hurt.

How old were you then?

I was nineteen, almost twenty. I came into A.A. when I was twenty-two. Towards the end I stopped going out with so many men. I was feeling so bad about myself. I was getting fat. I wasn't much fun to be around. I was more interested in spending time alone with food or girlfriends and going out in the evenings drinking.

I was seeking help during that time and I had tried Overeaters Anonymous. What I realize now is that I didn't think there was such a thing as having a male friend. I had this really bizarre idea that all you did with men was have sex with them. I don't know where I got that idea. Men were these people that were different and I was always attracted to them, but I was scared of them at the same time. In high school, my biggest fear was that I'd have to have sex with somebody. It was the last thing I ever wanted to do. In high school I had a fear that I'd become a drug addict. I had this tremendous fear that if I picked up a drug I'd never put it down. It must have been some kind of intuition; part of me knew that I was a compulsive person without ever having done a drug.

I always felt like I wasn't good enough or interesting enough. My parents have been married for forty years and they have a very good relationship. My sisters are married and they have healthy relationships with the men they married. So I don't know where I learned this really bizarre feeling about men. But I had it. My whole self-image was all wrapped up in my weight and how

I looked. Although God forbid, I would never admit that to any-body. I always acted as though I was very humble and could ac-cept anything about myself.

Was it fear of intimacy with men or were you afraid of being used?

It was intimacy. It was sharing how I felt and sharing my life that scared me. I never felt used. I was so terribly ashamed of what I was doing. I felt so worthless. I saw other people living and going to school, doing things they should be doing. Even though at times I was able to do those things, I did them half-assed. I was embarrassed to be a human being. I was just embarrassed to be alive. Everything about being a human being embarrassed me (laughs). It did.

Was there ever a period where you were really drinking a lot, too?

Yes. I had met this man that I seemed able to be friends with a little bit. It was the most I was ever able to talk to a guy really, and I loved it. He drank. He was an addict. He did a lot of coke. He did a lot of smoking dope. I didn't like it. Dope made me extremely paranoid, it made my throat swell up. I didn't like it, but I would do it occasionally. Occasionally I did some cocaine but I didn't really like that. I had no money, besides, so drinking was just the cheapest. I would prefer to use my money for food. With what money was left, I bought liquor.

The third time that I tried to be a college student was when I really started drinking a lot, every night. That went on for quite a few months. Then a friend mentioned to me that maybe I was having a bit of a problem with alcohol, and I said, "No, you're kidding. I'm a bulimic, I know what my problem is." We were out drinking one night with a couple of other friends and one night I remember being in the bathroom puking and puking and then trying to walk back out to the lounge where we were all sitting. I was drinking almost every day.

Alcohol changed my personality. It made me kind of funny and it made me mellow. But it also enabled me to do a lot of things that I never would have done had I not been drinking or bingeing—stealing money from people—to be able to keep up these habits. It was like I was a born thief. Like some kind of devil was putting these thoughts into my head. I was such a nice person. I was such an incredible people-pleaser that I really knew how to manipulate situations so that no one would ever suspect me. *Oh, sweet Hannah, she wouldn't do anything wrong.* When I think about some of the things that I've done, the stealing and the incredible lies I've told people I realize what a vicious cycle it was. The guilt led to drinking and more bingeing. It went around and around and around.

Obviously something made you decide enough is enough.

Well, it did. Like I said, even though I was into all of this drinking and bingeing I was seeking help. I was looking for a way out, and I had been for years. I had tried O.A. I had tried some therapy. I tried a number of self-help books, and nothing worked at all. I tried believing in a Higher Power. I tried believing that a power greater than me was going to save me from this and remove the obsession. And nothing did. I'd go to an O.A. meeting and then I'd come home and I'd binge or I'd drink. I would try therapy and I'd be bingeing before I went and I'd be telling them I hadn't been. I tried putting myself in school infirmaries for a couple of weeks at a time and nothing worked. By this time I had built up some relationships with some women in the O.A. program where I was living. I wasn't going any more but I still called them once in a while because I wasn't able to talk to any of my friends outside of the twelve-step program about what I was doing. They knew I had a problem but they had no idea what kind of hold it had on me—how it drove me to do things. I'd go to the bank and take out money that I didn't have, bouncing checks to go out and buy food. Then I'd go out to a bar later to drink. They had no idea I was doing this and I couldn't tell them because they just wouldn't understand. They wanted to see me get better. They felt sorry for me I think, but they couldn't help because they had no idea what they were dealing with, and I didn't either. I was in awe of how powerful this thing was—the obsession to drink and to binge like I did. It was just beyond me.

The last real drunk that I had had to do with a German woman I met in an O.A. meeting. She and her husband were going to Germany. She asked me to house-sit for her and I did. I realize now that I tried to kill myself in that apartment of hers. I locked myself in there for a couple of days. She had asked me not to drink any of their liquor. It was very, very expensive liquor that she and her husband had collected. She was not an alcoholic. I said fine, I won't. But I did. I also spent days in that apartment bingeing every free moment I had when I wasn't at work. At that point I was working two jobs. Just two retail jobs so they weren't too taxing. I didn't have to think much, and I could go in feeling awful and I frequently did. So I was there for a week in this apartment of hers. I lay on the bed, watched TV, drank wine, ate and threw up and ate and threw up and ate and threw up. I went out in the evening with some friends and drank myself to a point of being unable to walk. I was just a wreck. I felt so awful. It was time to go home, probably at about two in the morning. I had driven there myself. I stopped off to buy some food. I was so drunk that I could hardly walk or find the money to pay them. I ended up with a huge order of chicken. I started eating it the minute I walked out. I was eating and walking to my car, stuffing food in my face. I don't remember driving home. I have no idea how I got there. All I know is that I ended up in the apartment. I was still eating. I went into the bathroom and God knows what time it was, probably four in the morning by then and I had to go to work the next day at nine. But I wasn't thinking about that. I was thinking about throwing up. I went into the bathroom, still with food there. I knew that I had drunk enough liquid to make it easy to throw up. I hung over the toilet seat for an hour, maybe more. I had thrown up all over the floor, and by this time I had used up all of the paper in the house. There was no toilet paper, no paper towels, no Kleenex, nothing. I hadn't replaced any of the things that I had used all week long. I'd eaten all of their food. I was using towels to clean up the mess. I don't really remember. I was a wreck. I was half dressed and I was really scared because I thought I was going to die hanging over that toilet seat. That was one of the first times I realized that I might really die from this. People had told me I could. I managed to get up and go to bed. I fell asleep. I woke up around 9:30. I knew I was supposed to have been at work by 9:00. I didn't call. I tried to get up and I found that I couldn't. It was as if part of me was paralyzed. My left side was shaking and I couldn't bend my arms or walk. I got really frightened and started hyperventilating and crying and screaming. I didn't know what was happening. I was just really scared. I crawled over to the door of the apartment. I was still half dressed from whatever I'd had on the night before—I remember I had a little T-shirt on. I didn't have any pants on. I got myself over to the door but I wasn't able to open it because I was shaking so badly. It took me a while to realize that maybe I could use the other hand to open the door and get outside. I also had very bad pains in my stomach. I knew I needed help. I made it outside and up a couple of the steps to the people who lived upstairs. A woman came out. She took me upstairs. I was in so much pain. I was screaming, and unable to move. She said, "I'm taking you to the hospital." She got somebody to carry me into her car and she took me to the hospital, and she stayed there with me all day long.

They did all these tests. Basically I was fine. The doctor said I had eaten and thrown up so much food that there were some problems with my intestines. I had to take medication. This woman stayed there with me. And she said, "Don't worry, I won't tell this to anybody." She said, "When we're through here I'll take you back to Anna's apartment and I'll take care of you until they get back."

I took her up on her offer. She lived upstairs and fed me and pretty much took care of me. During that time I called a woman in O.A., and she said, "Have you ever thought that the way you're living is not normal? You're a twenty-two-year-old woman and you ought to be out living your life, not ending it." I guess I was ready to hear those words and have them mean something because that day I called up A.A. An old man answered the phone and he told me where there were some meetings.

I went to A.A. once a week for about a month. I knew I had a problem. I knew I was a bulimic. There was no question about that. I knew I was really sick in that area, but I didn't really believe I was an alcoholic. I was too young. How can a twenty-two-year-old be an alcoholic? That's what I kept asking myself and asking people at meetings. They just told me to keep coming back. During that month I went to one meeting a week, the same one, and oddly enough there was a man there who I thought was really cute. That kept me going back. He was nice. When I spoke up he responded, not as if to pick me up, but as a very adult, sober A.A. member. After a month of going once a week or so, I decided that I would do their 90 in 90.*

---

*Attend ninety meetings in ninety days.

The thing that really got me there was that people felt like I did. When I spoke up and shared whatever crazy thoughts were going through my mind people responded that they had felt the same way or they had thought the same thing. I sat there and I listened to what they were saying. I realized that, my God, they think like I do. I had never met anybody who really thought like I did—crazy, sick thoughts that I had. Even though I had had many close girlfriends, there were some things that I didn't share.

It's hard to explain, but there is a subtle difference in the way I thought as compared to the way my friends on the outside thought. But the key for me was that I put down the drink. I had one slip at about four months because I took a Valium and I didn't realize it was considered a slip. My sponsor said, "Technically that's a slip. I think we ought to change your sobriety date." So I did. It was my first year and I was still fairly skeptical of the program. I thought it was a brainwashing thing. I had a lot of thoughts about A.A., and whether or not I really belonged there. But the one thing I couldn't deny was that my life was getting better. I was bingeing less. I was not drinking.I had some real people that I could talk to about how I really felt. I could call my sponsor and she'd listen. And it could be all about me.

Did your weight level out?

Eventually it did. But what had to happen was I had to stop the throwing up. I didn't stop the bingeing right away. It tapered off to where I was doing it once a week, then once every couple of weeks, and then it was like once or twice a month, and I hit a plateau. I couldn't seem to make it without bingeing, but at least I was only doing it once or twice a month. And what people kept telling me was that they didn't care what I ate as long as I didn't throw it up. It took me a long time to get that concept. But slowly it came, and I would binge and I wouldn't throw up. I would sit with those uncomfortable, awful feelings. With all that food in me. What they were trying to teach me was that I had to learn to take the consequences of my actions. If I was going to eat that much food then I was going to gain weight and feel uncomfortable and live with it. And that philosophy worked for me. I was two and a half years into the program before I stopped my bingeing. But it had gotten very infrequent and it came up at times of stress.

When I was six months sober, I got involved with a married man in the program. I was still no saint. I absolutely fell madly in love with him. It was something I'd always looked for. He was wonderful. We were friends, we could talk. Yes, he was married and I felt bad about that. I'd always sworn I would never do anything like that, to hurt another woman like that, to be a part of the breakup of a marriage which was something that was so against what I believed in, but I did it anyway. I hope to God I never do anything like that again because it turned out to be a horrendous experience, very painful. The stress in that relationship is what sent me off bingeing. I began to see how stress-related the bingeing was. There were certain things that made me think of food and made it seem like a great escape.

If somebody asked you for advice, what would you say to them in terms of getting help?

I would say get yourself into A.A. Make some friends. Start talking about your feelings. Start working the twelve steps and begin learning how to love yourself. I would also say that some therapy would be a very good idea.

In the end, that's what it took for me with the bulimia. After my last binge and vomit session, my sponsor said, "Well, I think it's time that you get some professional help because you've been in the program for two and a half years. It's gotten much better but you're still bingeing. You need to address that." I went to see somebody for three or four months and that's when it stopped and I have not done it since.

The desire to do it has been removed. I don't want to do that to myself today. I rarely think about it. I can't say my weight is not important but it is not all-important today. I don't even think about it very much. I'm five feet two and I weigh about 118. My weight is fine. It has stabilized in the last year. When I came into A.A., I weighed about 140, maybe 145 from my bulimia and drinking . . . and slowly, about a year ago, I hit the 118 mark and I've been there ever since.

I never consciously tried to lose weight, not once. And I don't even know why because I had always tried to lose weight in the past. And now I believe it was a gift from my Higher Power. The obsession to lose weight and to figure out how much I was eating compared to how much I was burning up, all of that garbage that was occupying my mind about food and my weight . . . it was removed.

May 1990

Lucy

A drama professor at a university in the Midwest, she began recovering in Alcoholics Anonymous but stopped going to meetings after five years. She is fifty-six, five feet five, and thin. Her identity as an alcoholic is deeply enmeshed with her father's drinking. "My father was an alcoholic and when he got sober he did not go to A.A. That's interesting to me." She has two sons and although they are grown she still worries that her drinking may have harmed them. She stopped drinking on April 15, 1973, and this date still divides her life.

If you've noticed a bit of a reluctance about this, it comes from the fact that when I hear people say, "Yes, I drink too much. I'm going to go to a psychiatrist and I'm going to find out why I drink, then I'm going to be okay," I know that they're kidding themselves. I don't think getting to causes helps the problem, which is the addiction and the illness, but I don't know of anything out there that's better than A.A. I would always tell anyone out there who's in trouble to go to A.A. It's the only thing that we know works. And I believe that very fundamentally.

I went to my first A.A. meeting in ten years about a month ago. It was interesting because a woman whom I admire tremendously, a professional woman in the theater, in New York, was visiting in town and out it came that she'd been going to A.A. for a year. We were talking and she said, "I'd like so much to go to a meeting tonight, would you take me to one?" and I said, "Sure." So I took

her to one. There was supposed to be a non-smokers' meeting upstairs, and a smokers' one downstairs. The non-smokers' one had
not materialized. The room was blue. I could hardly breathe, being
an ex-smoker myself.

It was just so different from my last meeting. There was an enormous amount of cross-addiction, an enormous amount of drug addiction. I was quite turned off.

I think that the reason I drifted away from A.A. ten years ago—
I guess in a way in the very beginning, when I went and decided to
do something about it, I felt that *I* had done it. I didn't feel that I
had totally released myself to some sort of higher power. I had taken
action, and I was always sort of proud of my part in recovery. And
A.A. of course doesn't accept this. It's not what you do, so that was
the beginning of a bit of tension. Then in the group, I found that as
I got stronger, I needed it less. And then I found that there were
other women who were really troubled, who turned to me a lot and
I couldn't support that. I couldn't handle that. One of them who
had asked me to be her sponsor, and I had said I would, committed
suicide.

That devastated me. And I thought, "I can't be responsible." And
I also just felt a tremendous amount of guilt. That if I had given
her more, *now I'm not responsible*, but I always felt if I had given
more . . . .

As I got well, my career got wonderful, my relationship with my
husband, which had always been good, got better. My relationship
with our two sons, who were very little then, got better and I got
whole. And I didn't want . . . I didn't want to be associated with
cripples. And that really is why I pulled away. I don't know that
I've ever as fully articulated that because I could never fully articulate
that to someone in the program. They would detest me for saying
what I just said. Do you understand what I just said?

Yes.

I really believe that the statistics are pretty strong, you know,
there's a low recovery rate anyhow and yet A.A. has the highest
recovery rate. I guess what I would hope is that people . . . We had
a friend here who was very dear to me. He died as an old man, but
he bragged about the fact that he had been a Bowery bum. He was

a professor at the university. He went to a meeting every night of his life; he needed it. It was his opium, his alcohol, he went every single night and it was his life. I think that if he had ever stopped going to meetings he would have immediately started to drink again.

And I wonder if there are other women like us; people who aren't comfortable with A.A. And I guess I'm afraid that this could encourage people who really need the program, and who are recovering through the program, to drift away before they're ready. I'm still a little brainwashed.

Women in recovery exist outside of A.A. Women unable to grasp A.A. need to hear this.

Yes, to assuage my guilt. When I went to the meeting, a month ago, I did not know a soul. Not a soul. I couldn't believe it. Finally one woman came in that I had known, and I'm sure she looked at me and thought, "Lucy looks pretty good for someone who's been out there drunk for fifteen years. . . ." I mean, isn't that the assumption, if you're not there you're drunk? Because they teach you that if you move away from this program you will be drunk again. And that is not true. I not only don't drink, I think I'd rather pick up a cigarette first. I knew immediately that my life was so much better without alcohol.

I have a young friend, she's twenty-six—the daughter of one of my very dearest friends—and she has been struggling with drug addiction and alcohol for about six years, and she tries A.A. and she just can't make it. It breaks your heart.

Another thing I could never do in A.A. were twelve-step calls. They were too painful for me and I was afraid of being dragged back down. Somehow, partly because I'm an emotional person, I resisted that involvement. I resisted someone using me for their dependency. Someone needing to hang onto me terrifies me. It's a personal flaw in me. I would go and see a woman and she would need me and I would have to be a crutch for her, which I just did not want. Maybe I'm too selfish. I wanted to live my own life, to allow my positive energy to flow into things that were important to me. I guess I'm not big enough for that to have extended beyond my family, my husband, my work.

In the days when I was going to meetings, I never went to a

meeting without learning and gaining something. I never felt that it wasn't valuable. I was never bored. My discipline is theater. I teach theater and I'm also an actress and so I think the human interest of A.A. was very attractive to me. The stories, the emotions, the passion, the vulnerability, the fragility—all of those things fascinated me.

You'd be amazed how many actors and actresses are in A.A. It's incredible. I think it's a professional thing; you work at night and then you need to come down. It's hard to come down, after a rehearsal, or a performance. You're quite high. So you take alcohol to come down.

Do you want me to start from the beginning?

Yes.

My father was an alcoholic. He was a bender drinker. We would have great times and then he would go on a toot. He was very, very abusive, not physically abusive, verbally abusive. My brother was very clever, he would go to his room and shut the door, but I didn't do that. I would go into the fray and try to deal with it, which was stupid. My father, I think, was very fond of me, and the abuse turned particularly towards me. I've always wanted to please people, please the superior, please the adult, and I always think whenever anything goes wrong it's my fault. I carry a lot of the things that a child of an alcoholic carries.

I observed my father's drinking very carefully. I knew how he drank. I knew when he drank. I knew under what circumstances he drank. I could tell, by his face, if he'd had one drink. I got so sensitized to him.

My very first drinking experience—I was about fourteen, and I was doing a role in the local community theatre, playing the little sister in a play called *Dear Ruth.* The little girl gets drunk. It's a very funny scene. And one night I came home and I don't know if I was being a Stanislovsky actress or not, but I poured myself an orange juice glass full of bourbon and got drunk. It was just ghastly.

One of the things that characterized my drinking, through my drinking career, were the most unbelievably horrendous hangovers. That I would continue to drink with the kind of hangovers I had, amazes me. They were awful. But that was really the first time. And

I think it's fairly unusual that a fourteen-year-old kid would do that to herself.

Then I would enjoy a beer in high school. I dated a man who was older and we would go to bars. I would have a Tom Collins or a gin and tonic or something. But that was all okay. I did notice that alcohol changed my mood. I remember an occasion when a great aunt died, and I was asked to go to the funeral parlor and shake hands. I hated it and I was grumpy. But I went home with my family and had a couple of drinks, and that evening I was *wonderful*.

Either in late high school, or college, I realized that alcohol gave me something that as a human being I lacked. It gave me an ability to talk to people, to be charming, I *thought*. Maybe I wasn't at all. It gave me a social something that I didn't have. And there was a little man in the back of my head that said, "You're your father's daughter." Somehow I knew it and later in my drinking career it was as though I was programmed; I knew that's where I was going, I knew I was following in his footsteps. I almost seemed to be imitating him. That was a very curious thing and also a real awareness.

In college when I went to parties I drank a lot. I held it very well, and it gave me that freedom, that abandon that seemed to be wonderful. Right after college, I got a wonderful fellowship; a Woodrow Wilson fellowship, and I went to graduate school. I got a master's degree and I married my husband. I've been married to the same man for thirty-four years. I was almost twenty-three. I then went on to get my Ph.D.

That was a good, stable time. I didn't drink a whole lot. It was a very happy time. I was very active. Once in awhile, I would get drunk at a party. It was that pattern of compulsive behavior. They say if you're compulsive about food you can never eat that little dab of ice cream. When I started drinking, I drank until I was drunk. My husband and I liked martinis and we would often have a martini on a Friday or a Saturday before dinner, but everything was okay, everything was pretty stable for a long time.

After graduate school we went to a university in the Midwest and were there a couple of years. It was there that we had our first child. I was not working. After I got my Ph.D. we wanted to have a family. In those days it was appropriate for the husband to get the job, and the wife would just follow. If something turned up for me, all well and good. It was the beginning of a change in my whole attitude about life, and about myself. I had felt very good about myself as a graduate woman. All of a sudden I felt not very good about myself. I felt unworthy, unwanted, unneeded. We were very poor because my husband was a young professor. This was before our first baby was born. I had a job in a clothing store. I hated it. I took odd jobs. I was angry and bitter.

That was when the real drinking problem started, after our first son was born. I drank moderately when I was pregnant, which I have a lot of guilt about now, because we know some of the problems with that. I also smoked, and as you go on you worry about things.

Then we came here to Virginia, and once again I really didn't have a job. I was home with the baby. That was not the easiest thing for me, being home with the baby. I had a lot of trouble with that. We would go to parties and I can remember saying to myself, "Now I won't. I have such and such to do tomorrow. I can't face one of those horrendous hangovers." I had already talked to people about the nature of these hangovers.

There was one horrible occasion, when we were in Iowa and we'd been married a year—I got so drunk at a party one night that I began to flirt, pretty outrageously—I guess the word then was "necking"— with another man, pretty openly, in front of my husband. It was outrageous, and the next day I had a horrendous hangover, an incredible feeling of self-loathing. My husband was very angry. Rightfully so. That night is still something that's between us.

By the time our second son was born, I was maybe teaching an occasional course. But I was pretty much home with these two boys. I adored them but I wanted everything to be perfect. I wanted to be perfect Mom, and I rarely was. I wanted to be perfect everything. I think this is pretty typical alcoholic behavior. But I got very clever. I would greet George at the door with a beer to welcome him, so that he wouldn't know that I'd already had three, and then I started buying it, on the sly, to replace the supply. You know. The little devious things. There was a little man in my head saying, "You're your daddy's daughter."

There had been some terrible incidents, one was back in Iowa. There had been a party to welcome the new faculty and I got so drunk that I was just banging in the bathroom, flailing from wall to wall. That's pretty drunk. Somebody got me out of there. There I was, a new faculty wife with a husband just beginning his career, and I had to be literally carried out of this party. That made me just feel terrific. I would say, "Why do I do this? This is horrible behavior." When we came to Virginia, we've been here for twenty-five years, I would say that I was not going to drink too much at a party. The next thing I knew I would be lying in the bushes. Not all the time. But at parties or social situations it would just get awful.

The next step was buying vodka. I believed that myth that vodka doesn't smell on your breath. I would buy a bottle of vodka and keep it in my desk. I was working, I was functioning. I was directing a children's play at the university. I would lie down on the floor at the back of the theater and sleep. I was so drunk that I couldn't even function at my own rehearsal. But I fooled everybody; nobody even knew this. Everybody thought I was functioning. I think if you had asked my own husband he would have said, "She only drinks too much on occasion." I couldn't stop. I did outrageous stuff, yelling as my husband carried me out of the bushes. Screaming at my husband because he hadn't taken my contact lenses out of my eyes, things like that. We would go places and George would have a few drinks and say, "Gee, I don't think I'd better drive," and I would say, "I'll drive."

For years after I got sober, I had an incredible fear of driving because I was convinced that everybody on the road was drunk because I had driven drunk so many times. I remember our boys being involved in a Little League ball game. I drove seven children in a car on a Saturday afternoon when I was blind drunk. Hiding the vodka, I would sneak it into the house. It got so that once it was there I had a kind of serenity, a kind of peace knowing my stash was safely there. I didn't have to be drinking it. Just knowing it was there eased that terrible anxiety when I didn't have anything in the house.

If I was drinking, I was waking up at four o'clock in the morning with the sweats and then the dry heaves. Hangovers, there was no cure for them. They would last the whole next day. Of course my parents had taught me that there was one good cure for a hangover: start drinking again. I guess in A.A. they would call me a high bottom drunk.

I kept having this recurring nightmare. I was in the bottom of a black pit and I kept trying to claw my way out of it, but I couldn't. I would slide in this mud, back down into the pit. Then I would try to claw my way up, and I would slide back down. This nightmare began to pervade my whole life. I had blackouts. My husband would tell me of things I had done. I had no memory of them.

I began to abuse the children. I would grab their arms and get extremely authoritarian and very angry, which is not my nature at all. I'm a pretty gentle person. And then I would hate myself.

The summer before I stopped drinking we went to Indiana. Presumably we were working on a book. We didn't get any work done. My husband's family was out there and one of his brothers was a big drinker. I just used that as an excuse for that summer to be one prolonged party. We went to the liquor store every day. By this time I was drinking heavily every night, sometimes passing out at eight or nine o'clock. The rest of them went on normally.

My husband was a saint. He didn't say anything. He had to travel a good deal at that point. I would buy gallons of cheap chablis. By then I had started teaching part time. I had a lot of anger about that because I was very conscientious, and worked very hard, but I was only a temporary part-time instructor. My whole career was on hold.

One night I called a man that I knew in A.A. I remember him saying, "This is the first night of the rest of your life," or some bullshit like that. I thought, "Oh Jesus." But I did make that call. He said that he would have a woman in the program get in touch with me.

Well, I thought everybody was going to stand on their head for me, and treat me like the queen bee, and fuss over this brilliant woman, who was now a drunk. Well, they didn't at all, but the woman called me. She was a professor at the university and has since died. She became my sponsor. She was the most wonderful, intelligent woman. She was the single most important thing in A.A. for me. I admired her mind, I admired her talent, I admired everything about her. She was simply wonderful. She wrestled and had several slips. But I do not think that her death was alcohol related.

She took me to a meeting. It was on a Monday night. Another woman went to the meeting, another local woman. The other woman was very articulate. She talked about pulling the shades and drinking after her children went to school. I was so affected that when it came my turn, I didn't say a word, I just wept. Later they told me that they put their money on the one who cried, rather than the one who talked.

I loved it and I, immediately, overnight, was better. Overnight, the cloud lifted. That nightmare lifted. I started sleeping better. I went on a euphoric high that was incredible.

Because I had felt so used by the university, throughout all this temporary part-time teaching shit that had gone on for years, I resigned. And I had no sooner resigned than they offered me a contract, as a full-time assistant professor. I'm now a full professor, with all rights and privileges. To this day, I mark things in my life as before April 15 or after April 15, 1973.

Everything just started to turn around, and it was all associated with that point of sobriety. I began to realize that I had tremendous resentments, tremendous anger, tremendous inner rage. And I think a lot of it was about being a woman, about being an educated woman, an *unemployed*, educated woman. All of that turned around too. And I have to tell you that I have been treated very, very well by this university. I moved along, and have been a full professor now for a number of years. Everything just got better.

You would be surprised how many alcoholic graduate students appear. I can look at someone and know the person is having a problem with alcohol. I can spot it easily. I've been able to help a number of graduate students. I don't blab it, it's not common knowledge, but I do tell people about my history. When I tell them, I tell them it was A.A. that worked for me. I had tried to stop before, or to control my drinking, and I'd have luck for a little while. Just long enough to fool myself. And I would drink again, exhibiting all the same behavior as my father. I knew it, I recognized it, and I think I ultimately knew I was going to do something about it.

My father died sober. He did not use A.A. That's very interesting to me. He did not use A.A. and the last four years of his life he was totally sober. He quit on his own. But when I told my mother she wept, and asked me, how had she failed me, why had my life gone wrong? I tried to explain that it had nothing to do with her, that it probably was, to a large extent, genetic.

I sense the pain of these kids who are in trouble with alcohol. I try to help them. Without prying, or pushing, I'll talk to anyone about it if they're interested, or if it comes up naturally, in a conversation. We had some friends for dinner recently and I began to talk about drinking and family members, and how it touches many lives. Everybody in this country has the pain of alcoholism somewhere in their lives. My husband's life was damm near destroyed. His father and then his mother began to drink.

I worry about our sons. When they were growing up I tried to get them to go to an A.A. meeting with me. I tried to get them interested. They totally rejected it. And I thought, in a way, it might have been better if they hadn't been so young when I got sober and had experienced a little bit of the pain of it. They both drink. I don't see any problems emerging yet, but I have told them that there is a family history, and they need to be sensitive to that. I've told them that if ever they do have a problem to remember that A.A. is the place to go.

What A.A. is in basic theory is getting out of the self. Reaching out to somebody else, doing something outside the self. That's what the program is all about. Admitting it, and that's such a hard step, admitting it. But when you do it's like a great burden has been lifted from your shoulders.

Remembering some of the things I did, like drinking the kirsch for fondue, or putting the beer can in a towel so that George wouldn't hear the pop of the tab opening, is good. Being aware of the devious things I would do, I'm not a devious person, but remembering these things has been a good thing to do. . . .

I've never had a slip. I will put a little Amaretto or crème de menthe on top of ice cream, but I don't think of that as drinking. I cook with wine. There's been alcohol in the house from the day I stopped drinking. I knew that our social life would not change, and the thing, of course, that amazed me immediately was how little others drink. I thought everyone drank as much as I did. They don't.

We went to a dinner party. I had been sober for a week or two. There was a man who worked for the *New York Times* who sat next to me at dinner. I put my hand over my wineglass as they were serving the wine. He said, "How do you get through the day without a drink?" and I whispered to him, "My problem was getting through a day *with* a drink." And he said, "Oh." But I am amazed that I put my hand over a wineglass; no one ever pushes or forces drinks. . . .

When I first stopped drinking, I'd order a Perrier or a cranberry juice, and they'd bring the damn thing in an orange juice glass. I now say, "In a pretty glass, please." In a beautiful glass, that's a part of it. I have a dear friend who has wonderful blown-glass goblets and he always gives me my Perrier or my club soda, which is what I really prefer, with a nice twist of lime, in this beautiful blown-glass goblet. I just love it.

I use a lot of things in A.A. I use the Serenity Prayer. I use it a lot because I realize that one of my biggest problems was my "Oh gosh, I've got this to do, and this to do, and on and on." I say one day at a time, "You have *this* to do. Forget the rest. Get through this."

I say to my husband, *"God grant me the serenity to accept the things I cannot change, the courage to change the things I can, and the wisdom to know the difference."* That's wonderful advice. Absolutely wonderful advice.

A.A. is really exactly like Christianity or Buddhism or Confucianism. Good religions that work for people have these common bases, these common themes and ideologies. So much of A.A. is good common sense, just good philosophy.

February 1990

Marty Mann

Marty Mann was born in 1904. Striking, with blue eyes and short brown hair, she was the first woman to recover in Alcoholics Anonymous. Four years after Bill Wilson and Dr. Bob Smith created A.A., it consisted of approximately fifty men. Lois Wilson, Bill's wife, started Al-Anon, the program for nonalcoholic wives. Nice women from good backgrounds were not expected to become alcoholics. They were shunned, and Marty Mann was no exception. She always had the support of Bill Wilson, however, and with that, she was finally accepted into A.A. She spent the rest of her life helping other alcoholics. She was one of the first women to begin hacking away at the stigma surrounding women who drink too much. She founded the National Council on Alcoholism. Her book New Primer on Alcoholism *is still considered a classic. Jane, who told me Marty's story, said, "No book about women in recovery would be complete without Marty Mann's story, for it was she who paved the way for the rest of us." Marty was Jane's sponsor from 1969 up until Marty's death in 1980.*

As most of us do when we first come into the program, I steeped myself in the lore and literature available on the subject of alcoholism. And of course I'd heard of Marty Mann, the first woman to recover in Alcoholics Anonymous. I would see her at Bill Wilson's big dinners, held every fall in New York. They took place in a grand hotel ballroom, attracting alcoholics from all over. They ran like big, open meetings. Bill would tell his story, and Marty would be sitting up there on the dais with Lois. Marty was a figure of some controversy among some of the old-timers who felt that she had founded the National Council on Alcoholism to further her own fame and fortune. Which, in my view, couldn't have been further from the truth. Bill Wilson was a big, tall, spare Yankee, not a charismatic speaker. But Marty was very charismatic. She was a fabulous speaker.

The first thing she would say about herself, even in public, was, "I am a recovering alcoholic." Well, you can imagine. It was like a nuclear bomb going off. A lot of people were horrified. "Oh, how can she do that?" It caused her serious problems; the alcoholic stigma was so strong. For instance, in 1954 she was engaged in a lawsuit against an airline. Those were the days when even the big planes landed in the open and you walked down the steps. She fell, and there was a lawsuit with the airline because their contention was she fell because she was drunk, even though she'd been sober for about twenty years. She didn't back off. Marty never backed off from anything; she was a woman of great conviction. So of course, I would see her, never dreaming that one day she would become my sponsor and close friend.

I would sit there at Bill's dinners thinking, "Wow, there's Bill. Wow, there's Marty Mann." And then, once in awhile, "There's Lois." Because Lois had created Al-Anon and was Bill's wife. I held her in esteem and awe but not to the degree that I thought of Bill and Marty.

I didn't know Lois well. I met her at Marty's memorial service and she couldn't have been sweeter. During the eulogy, which a young assistant minister conducted at the Congregational Church in Westport, it sounded as though he really knew her quite well. At one point in Marty's life, which I'll get to later, she had been given the manuscript of the Big Book of A.A. and had thrown it out. I didn't tell the minister that Marty had rejected it because she was so horrified by the constant appearance of the word God. By her own admission, she said, at that point in time, that she was an intellectual; she had given up the notion of God at the age of seventeen. And so she hurled the whole thing out the window . But during the service, Lois piped up and said, as the minister was describing Marty reading the manuscript of the Big Book, "Yes. She threw it out the window." And everyone laughed.

Marty was one of four children born to a prominent Chicago family. When she was fourteen, she contracted tuberculosis and was sent out to a sanatorium in Arizona. It was during a crucial time in her development. Adolescence, even for Marty Mann I'm sure, was difficult. Perhaps more so because she was isolated as an adolescent. I guess that's where she became withdrawn and shy. She'd lost contact with all her friends, all her peers. Prior to going West, she had been a very precocious child, intelligent with a very keen wit. She thought nothing of ignoring the rules and roles set down for girls in the early part of the century. She was restless and energetic all her life and was evidently often at odds with her father. She would also say, "I was the bane of my gentle mother's existence." All of this was tempered by the long and pretty serious bout with tuberculosis which separated her from her family for the long convalescence. She was seventeen when she returned to Chicago and she had turned from a gregarious child into a very serious and withdrawn young woman.

Things had changed during her absence. It was 1922. Prohibition had spawned the greatest drinking spree in history. And as she tried to make the awkward reentry into the family and social circles, she discovered that after the years of semi-isolation, she'd lost the ability to relax and converse with people. She'd become extremely shy and as she described it, "tongue-tied." So she went from being willful and gregarious to feeling awkward and inarticulate. "Drinking was all around," she said. "Every boy I went on a date with had a silver flask in his hip pocket. I was offered drinks, and found they metamorphosed me into my old self. Drinking was an important part of everyone's social life, whatever age they were, and I saw nothing unusual about that. It was just the way life was. If you didn't drink, you weren't asked on dates." She quickly discovered that one, two, or three drinks untied her tongue and she could do the Charleston and the Black-Bottom as well as everyone else at all the lavish debutante parties she went to at the mansions on Lake Shore Drive. But best of all, and this is the way she described it, "Drinks untied my tongue. Nobody had to force bathtub gin or champagne on me. I loved it. I liked it very much." And that's when she discovered she had this enormous capacity. At one party there was another girl, named Virginia as she recalled, also noted for her great capacity for alcohol. The boys decided they'd have a competition to see who could drink whom under the table. It started with everybody drinking bathtub gin, or no, French 76.

That's champagne and brandy?

Yes, champagne and brandy. You know, real dynamite. I mean, you could launch a rocket to the moon with that. And so she and Virginia began drinking; all the boys were drinking. As the evening progressed and she and Virginia went on, seemingly unaffected, "One by one," she said, "the boys would literally drop out. They would drop to the floor. By dawn, Virginia and I and three boys judging the contest, who were not drinking, were the only ones still on our feet." She said the room was just filled with these humps where people had dropped in their evening clothes. So they decided to go out and make a big party of breakfast. And the decision was that it was a draw. She had no doubt, years later, that Virginia was probably an alcoholic, too, because she drank the same way Marty did. But it wasn't until she was sober that she realized that.

Meanwhile, she got married. It was a wild, drunken spree. That's what many young women did. I gather that her husband was also an alcoholic. The marriage was short-lived; she was very restless and unhappy and not at all cut out for the role of being the good wife and mother and all of that. She wanted more. She always felt the world had more to offer and she wanted to find out about it.

She decided to go to London because her feeling was that photojournalism, which was what she wanted to go into, was a field dominated by men. She decided to go to London where the attitudes, strangely enough—when you think of England today—were much more receptive to creative women than they were in Chicago. She opened her own studio. By this time she was very tall, with piercing blue eyes and a very dry wit oiled by booze. She soon became the darling of the literati and the Shaftesbury Avenue crowd.

Was she a good photojournalist?

Yes, she was. She was twenty years old and a woman of broad interests, free to do anything she wished. Her family didn't stand in her way; they encouraged her to be all that she could be. They were probably distressed by her drinking. Her mother particularly, because she felt it wasn't ladylike to drink at all, let alone drink the way Marty did. In the beginning, her alcoholism, which was certainly taking shape, wasn't recognized as such by her new brilliant circle of friends. They just simply did what a lot of people probably still do today with people in the arts: they attributed her behavior to her creative genius. It was the thinking that all artists are a little mad. So as her behavior gradually became bizarre, it was not only condoned but encouraged.

Do you think that's still true today?

Yes, definitely. It's unfortunate. I mean, with all that's known of the disease, there are still people who really don't know. People of great intelligence who you would think *should* know. Anyway, she was hanging out with well-known artists and writers of the day, spending the summer in the south of France with people like Jean Cocteau and Picasso. The twenties were a wonderful time in life and in history. Everything was in a state of change, anything was possible. It was a time of experimentation and throwing out of all the old rules. They were all young and talented and blessed with extraordinary constitutions. And as she said, "Some of them actually were mad."

When she was twenty-seven, in 1931, everything changed. That's when alcohol took over her life. Now she was experiencing terrifying blackouts and starting to see doctors, none of whom could explain the cause of the blackouts. She became convinced she was going mad. At that point she met two guys who were running a fifteenth-century Jacobean inn in a little village in the Cotswolds called Broadway. The owners went off to Spain for the winter leaving Marty to run things. It was hunt country and she loved to fox hunt. Of course, when you fox hunt, you start off with a snort. A lot of people get killed fox hunting probably because they had a few brandies too many before they set out. Anyway, there she was in this setting that looked like a picture book: this beautiful inn, this beautiful country. But restless as ever, one day she started exploring the inn and she went up into the attic and there was this enormous stash of dandelion wine which had been put up there to age. She proceeded to systematically drink it all through the winter. When the owners of the inn returned, they began to hear questionable things about Marty's behavior, not only from the guests but from some of the townspeople.

Then they discovered all the dandelion wine missing. They confronted her and she left the inn and returned to London in a state of
high dudgeon, you know, the way we always do. No one had ever
spoken to her like that and she wouldn't tolerate it. So, ill as she
was, she resumed the photography. She was, miraculously, still able
to handle the camera with skill.

The following summer, a Fourth of July party was held for Amer-
icans and for friends that were coming home. Marty disappeared
early and was found sometime later on the terrace—in pieces. She'd
fallen from a window. Years later, in the last years of her life, she
told me, "I said I'd fallen, but I really jumped." Her leg was fractured
near the hip, her jaw was fractured on both sides, all her lower teeth
had been knocked out, and she'd bitten off the sides of her tongue.
She was rushed to a nearby hospital where she was kept in agony
for five days before being moved to the orthopedic hospital in London. And for the next six months she was in traction with an eight-
pound weight pulling her leg back to its normal length. Of course,
she spent the whole time in the hospital drinking.

How did she get alcohol in a hospital?

Friends brought it to her. All her writer, actor, and artist friends
would all come in to see her bringing her whatever she wanted. Gin,
wine, champagne; whatever she wanted. Again, alcoholism wasn't
treated as a disease, it was still very much under, you know, it still
had the mystery, the myth that nice people weren't alcoholics. Especially nice women from nice families. So her friends would come
in and regale her with stories of what was going on in London and
they'd drink. Plus, morphine was the only pain killer in the hospital.
So there she was with the morphine and the booze. During the down
times, when she had no visitors, she'd lie there immobile, pondering
her life and her sanity. She was convinced she was losing her mind.
Even though she'd never been in a mental institution, she had a great
fear of them.

Do you think that runs in alcoholics, a fear of mental hospitals?

Yes. Because anyone who is an alcoholic knows the insanity of
the disease, knows it as a very real and viable fear. So she decided

as soon as she was able to walk again, that she'd return to the United States and go mad here. The feeling was that if she had to be institutionalized, she'd rather be in America where at least she had family and some friends left. During the time she was in the orthopedic hospital in traction, she befriended a young nurse who was from Scotland and evidently very much in love with a young man back in her village. Marty encouraged her to go back to Scotland and marry him. Which the nurse did. And they corresponded.

Virtually without money when the time came for her to leave the hospital, the young nurse invited Marty up to convalesce in her home in the north of Scotland, near Inverness. It's very beautiful country—magical, mystical, very rugged and very poor. Up there she learned to walk again, first with crutches, then with a cane, and finally unassisted and without a limp. She would always mention that the name of this couple, Skinner, was appropriate because that was the groom's trade: he trapped and skinned rabbits, which were a prime source of meat in the U.K. then. And so, to pay her way, Marty began the next stage of her life as a trapper. She went out and trapped rabbits. That's how she survived. Another reason that motivated her to accept the invitation was that she knew she wouldn't be able to drink up there. The Skinners lived very simply and whiskey was a luxury they just couldn't afford. But this wasn't the case at the parties that were held in the village. There she drank a lot of whiskey. Taught the villagers all the American dances and cowboy yells that she'd learned after all those years in Arizona while recovering from TB.

While she was in Scotland, Marty read *Asylum* by William Seabrook. Now she had known Seabrook in the states. They used to drink together. He had apparently gone to a hospital, undergone extraordinary treatment, and emerged able to drink again. Marty wanted that too, not in the least bit put off by the vivid descriptions of Seabrook trussed up in wet sheets and held under hot and cold running water. She wanted anything that would enable her to drink. So she decided that she would go back to the United States and go through this treatment so that she could drink "normally" again. She began concentrating on saving and conniving enough money for her return passage. She sailed home from England determined not to drink. It was 1938 and clouds of war were looming on the horizon. She decided not to drink during the voyage. She was really going to make a new start. How many times have we all said that? The other good thing, what she felt very optimistic about, was that no one in New York knew the bizarre turn her life had taken in England, so she'd be free. She'd be able to start over again and that was her thought as she boarded the ship. And then, as she'd say in her story, "I didn't see the Statue of Liberty, the New York skyline, in fact, I didn't even know we had arrived. I didn't walk off the ship, I was carried off on a stretcher and delivered to my sister and mother who were waiting on the pier, whom I had not seen for seven years." In those days when you crossed an ocean there was nothing but one long party. I mean, you drink morning, noon, and night. And because she was attractive, witty, and bright, and because she didn't have the insight yet to realize that the only way she could cope with groups of people was to drink—she drank. That insight didn't come until much later.

Broke and unemployable, she was "treated" by friends to a visit with Dr. Foster Kennedy, a leading neurologist. She thought her friends were also alcoholics, not doing anything about their drinking. But they weren't having the kinds of dreadful problems Marty was having. They said, "Why don't you go see Dr. Kennedy?" She said, "All right." She really was terrified that she was losing her mind. And so she went to see Kennedy and he assured her that she was not insane. He did agree to take her into his neurological ward at Bellevue because she was so obviously ill. And it was at this time that she understood the full meaning of the phrase—and she always had this in her story—"people like you." You know. She'd heard that many times, from baffled physicians who could not diagnose what was wrong with her, nor offer her any solution to her rapidly deteriorating health. What Kennedy said to her was, "In my experience, people like you rarely survive. Those that do are one in a million. Because you want to get well so badly, I'm going to take a chance that you're that one." He admitted her to the neurological ward, saw her briefly every day, and murmured sympathetically when she told him that what she was getting in the way of treatment was just an illusion, that she needed something more. She kept saying that to him. "I need something else. I need something more." And he'd shake his head and say, "Well, this is all we have." Finally, after nearly a year, he arranged Marty's transfer to Blythewood, a magnificent psychiatric treatment facility in Connecticut situated on the old Boss Tweed estate. It was a huge country home sprawling over five hundred acres in Greenwich. The facility was run by Dr. Harry M. Tiebout. It was Tiebout who suggested to Marty that her illness might have a connection with alcohol and that if she didn't drink at all she might be able to resume a normal life. So she tried not to drink much of the time at Blythewood. But every now and then, for reasons no one could explain, and after long periods of good behavior, she drank. She got weekend passes to go to New York, to the theater, or to the dentist—she'd go in sometimes and she'd be fine, and come back without having picked up a drink. But other times she would go in and she drank. She'd come back drunk. Tiebout finally put her on a warning, after she'd been in Blythewood for almost two years, that one more drunken episode and that was it, she'd be out the door. She really had no money, nowhere to go. These people who had taken her in obviously thought enough of her to try and help her. And there was Kennedy thinking she might be that one in a million who could make it.

After two years she knew the staff quite well and they all liked her, so she still continued the pattern. She'd go to New York, sometimes without a drink, and sometimes she'd get drunk. When she came back drunk the staff would whisk her out of sight and try all the sobering up cures: putting her in showers, giving her coffee, and all of this. Well, one weekend after she came back drunk she got a summons to Tiebout's residence. He was in bed with the flu, and Marty was convinced that this was it, he was calling her in to give her her walking papers. She'd been drunk the previous weekend. She had no money and no place to live. As she approached the bed timidly, Tiebout was motioning to a chair excitedly, and to a manuscript bound in a red cardboard that was resting on the coverlet. He said, "Marty, I've got it! I've got something written by people like you. I want you to take it to your room and read it." And of course the manuscript was the book *Alcoholics Anonymous*. It was being submitted to members of the clergy and the medical profession prior to publication. Bill and Bob didn't want to offend anyone in those areas and so anyone they could think of was given a manuscript to read to make sure they weren't going to say anything that would create any problems. Marty took the manuscript back to her room and tentatively opened the red cover. At first when she started to read, she was electrified. Teibout was right. She did have a lot in common with these people. Then she threw the book to the floor in disgust, and this is a direct quote: "Nowhere had I seen the word God so many times on a written page. I couldn't believe Tiebout would give me such tripe. I was an intellectual. I had given up God when I was seventeen." And she told Tiebout as much at their next meeting. He said that nonetheless, he wanted her to keep on reading, which she did, forcing herself to read just enough pages to get through the next quiz with Tiebout. She said that the other thing that really bothered her was that nowhere, and this is another direct quote, "Nowhere did the book mention women. I was convinced that these poor benighted people were deluded, suffering from self-hypnosis, and I told Tiebout so." See, nothing's new.

Tiebout said he really would like her to go to New York and meet some of the men who had written this book. "I balked," Marty said, "for about three months. It wasn't that I had a problem with accepting the fact that I was an alcoholic, that I had a disease called alcoholism. I was happy to have those words. You would be too if you had been a nonentity as long as I was. I just didn't see what good meeting these other alcoholics would do and they were probably a seedy lot anyway." And so she wouldn't go. Their meetings from then on were spent with Tiebout trying to get her to go and her balking. But finally, after three months, she gave in. Tiebout handed her a card with an address on Sutton Place, which wasn't so bad. When she got there she found the host was a charming Virginian gentleman who had arranged a handsome dinner partner for her. "It was lovely and no one said anything upsetting to me, and the host was a man named Popsy Maher." Popsy was one of the earliest members of A.A. After this lovely dinner, with no booze, Popsy said, "All right, it's time," whereupon they headed for the subway and the long ride to Brooklyn Heights, where the meetings were held in those days. This was 1939, when there were less than fifty members of Alcoholics Anonymous holding a meeting every Tuesday at the Wilson's house. There were no women. "All during the subway ride, men joined us, carrying their worldly possessions in brown paper bags. They were more in keeping with what I expected an alcoholic to look like—destitute, in shapeless clothes."

"Bill's house was on a nice quiet street. As soon as we were in Brooklyn Heights, as soon as we entered, I knew, I just knew, I couldn't go in there. That had been the trouble all along. All my life I had needed a drink in order to meet new people. How could I possibly do something as important as this without a drink?" So she fled to the bedroom where the coats were being kept and flung herself on top of them, weeping. Eventually a woman came in and sat down beside her and placed her hand gently on Marty's shoulder and she

said, "Please come in. We've been waiting for you for a very, very
long time." Of course, the woman was Lois, Bill's wife. She herself
was not an alcoholic, but had lived with Bill's alcoholism for so long,
she became as much a sponsor to Marty as Bill was. "She was the
only woman for me to talk to for the longest while."

Marty was finally released from Blythewood and she returned to
New York and attended the Tuesday meetings regularly. The men
who were in the group thought she was a freak: that there really was
no such thing as a woman alcoholic.

Why did they think women couldn't be alcoholics?

Drinking was really something that men did and nice women did
not do. So the women were driven underground. They were hidden
and while I'm sure that women drank all along, they hid it well.
They drank at home. They would sober up before the men came
home. And everyone believed that only the lowest of the low, slat-
terns and whores drank. Nice women from good families didn't
drink. But Bill knew better because he and Bob had tried to help a
woman out in Akron, and before that there'd been another woman
who I believe was from Washington, D.C. But she had come briefly
and then left and never came back, and no one knew what had become
of her.

*But Marty was the one who made sure that women got some help. Didn't
she go to Dorothy Parker and other women . . . ?*

Oh yes, through the council she tried to help tremendous numbers
of women. I mean, they're legion, but in these early meetings, at
the house in Brooklyn Heights, the men in the group really felt that
there was no such thing as a woman alcoholic. They were, in other
words, the exception, not the rule. They weren't saying a woman
couldn't be an alcoholic, just that they were real oddities. Marty said,
"I decided I didn't care what happened. I was still broke, without a
decent job. I decided to stay in A.A. no matter what." She kept
going to the meetings, but I guess with all their hammering at her
and with their doubting, she decided what the hell. She holed up in
a friend's apartment, where she thought no one could find her. She

said, "I was going to drink. Nothing else mattered. Bill and Lois had lost their house in foreclosure. Everyone in A.A. seemed to be a loser, God knows I was a loser and couldn't bear it. I was coming back from the liquor store with my supply of bottles, and there was Bill, standing in the little foyer of the apartment building, peering at all the names on the mailboxes. I was in a rage, I was furious, I had no idea how he had found me and he had no business interfering in my life and I told him as much. He was a tall and gaunt man with his thin wrists hanging out of an awful-looking raincoat. As soon as he saw me I told him he wasn't going to stop me. I was still clutching my bag, my bottles of booze. He said, 'All right.' But first he wanted to talk to me so I reluctantly let him in." The group, Bill explained, had done a 180-degree turn and had decided Marty was indeed an alcoholic, and they had donated money to pay for Marty's hospitalization at Towns Hospital, which was then the only hospital in New York that would admit an alcoholic. So Marty said, "The sight of all those rumpled ones and fives being pulled from Bill's pockets was more than I could bear, and I turned away and told him I couldn't accept their money."

It was winter, and Bill and Lois were living in an unheated cabin that someone in the fellowship had loaned them. Bill asked Marty if she would consider coming home with him, that he and Lois would try and nurse her back to health. So she said she would do that. But after several weeks of intensely severe winter weather in a summer cabin where you could see the daylight through the walls, she had to be hospitalized. In the next forty-one years, she never drank again.

As her recovery began, she would regain the use of her mind and her eloquent tongue. She fought tirelessly to educate the world about the disease of alcoholism. I never observed her breaking her anonymity—but she did say that she was a recovering alcoholic. She founded the National Council on Alcoholism, primarily to create a platform from which she could go public and spread the disease concept. Alcoholism was, for a long period, called Jellinek's disease, named for the doctor who founded the School of Yale Studies on the subject. He held seminars for two summers in the forties. His most famous book is *The Disease Concept of Alcoholism*. Marty participated in those seminars.

It was then that Bill and Marty began to try to get the American Medical Association to define alcoholism as a disease. Even today, people have problems with that concept. Marty used the council as a platform where she could educate not only the public but the medical profession, that alcoholism was indeed a disease, that it was nothing to be ashamed of. She stood up and said this. The statement was outrageous at the time, and it flew around the world on all the wire services.

Did she start believing in God, or in a Higher Power?

She believed in God.

Marty took on the courts, again using the council as a platform, admonishing judges for sentencing alcoholics to drunk tanks. She'd say, "Imagine the hue and cry if this were done to epileptics suffering from grand mal seizures. Alcoholism is the same thing." Her book, *Marty Mann's New Primer on Alcoholism,* is still considered a classic in the field.

In the fifties, the estimates were that one out of every six alcoholics was a woman, and by the seventies, it was one woman for every four men. Marty always believed that this data was understated simply because women didn't stand the same scrutiny. And that they were harder to ferret out. And as we well know today, as Marty always believed from the beginning, the ratio is equal.

And during the primary years, the early years of the council, she was subject to ridicule and contempt by many members of A.A., who felt that what she was doing was out of hand and out of line. But many a well-known woman alcoholic, and many women who never recovered, Dorothy Parker being one, came through the council offices and Marty was tireless in her efforts to help them, to explain the disease concept, and of course her prescription was always A.A.

She often suffered long and intensive bouts of depression, right up until the end of her life. She had that battle to contend with, and she had throat cancer which fortunately was caught very early. She had surgery for that.

Marty Mann devoted her life to educating the public about alcoholism. After she finally retired from the Council, she would still go in for board meetings. A few months before she died I asked her whether people flocked to her the way they did Bill. "Do they all bow and salaam when you walk down the hall?" And she looked at me with this twinkle in her eye and said, "Hell no, they don't even know who I am. No, thank God, they don't do that." She was also working regularly at Silver Hill down in New Canaan where she ran the alcoholic treatment facility in the last years of her life. The idea of Marty sitting around and not doing anything, even though she was seventy-four, was absurd. She was still going to meetings every day, or practically every day; I think she went five days a week. She never gave up on anyone that she worked with. I mean, people who were full of denial and anger, she never gave up on them. She was very patient and she'd cut right through the bullshit with people. She wasn't afraid to tell you what was really going on.

Wasn't she the first person to come up with the idea that anger is what we can't afford?

Well, back when she was reading the manuscript, during the Blythewood stay, after she had thrown the first draft of the Big Book out the window because of her revulsion at the mention of God on every page, she'd gone to New York and she'd had a drink. Something had happened to someone she was very fond of and she was very angry at the person who had victimized her friend. So she picked up a drink, you know, she drank at the situation. She used to say, "What we do when we're angry is we look around for the biggest mallet we can find and bang ourselves over the head with it. And if it isn't booze, we'll find something else, even in sobriety." She felt that—she got back to her room and knew she was going to have to see Tiebout. She picked up the manuscript which was, by then pretty battered, and she started to read. "You know the expression 'seeing red'? I always thought it was just a metaphor, just A.A. rhetoric. I didn't realize that you actually could see red. I saw red when I saw the word God. But there on the page, where it says we cannot afford anger, the words were clear and in white. I felt that was the beginning of my spiritual awakening." It was after that that she agreed to go and meet Bill Wilson.

That's in her story in the Big Book.[*]

Yes. You can fill in the blanks with that. Marty lectured daily. As time went on, she realized she was not getting to A.A. meetings.

[*]*Marty's story appears in the second edition, published in 1955.*

She was becoming, as she said, "A professional alcoholic." And she would speak on the subject of alcohol for years and years. Then her health began to fail; she couldn't maintain that schedule, but she literally did it anyway, if not 365 days a year, darn close. It dawned on her that she wasn't getting any A.A., that she was spending all of her time flying all over the world talking about alcoholism but not listening.

In 1943, Dr. E.M. Jellinek of Yale came to A.A. and said to Bill, "Yale, as you know, is sponsoring a program on public education on alcoholism, entirely noncontroversial in character, and we need, or we'd like the cooperation of A.A. to proceed with unending education projects concerned with alcoholism." To Jellinek, proceeding without the cooperation of A.A. would be unthinkable. So Marty went up to Yale that summer, and then Bill went up and did the final talk.

Meanwhile, *The Cleveland Plain Dealer* assigned a writer named Albert Davis to cover A.A. and go the limit. So for days on end articles about A.A. in general and about A.A. in Cleveland in particular, were featured in *The Cleveland Plain Dealer*. Beside these articles there appeared editorials which said, "A.A. is good. It works, come and get it." And there was a huge deluge. So Bill, Marty and Lois piled into a car and drove out to Cleveland to see what was going on. That was when Marty got up and spoke, looking around the room—there were about a hundred people—no one had ever seen that many people in one A.A. meeting. Overwhelmed, she said, "Wouldn't it be great if someday there were rooms like this all over the country." And everyone laughed. What a grandiose alcoholic thing to think! I mean the idea of a world concept was beyond their imaginations at that point in time.

What is so great is that the weekend before her death, she had been down at the big A.A. convention in New Orleans and was very excited when she came back because the flags of thirty-five nations were represented there, and of course, because she had spoken. She had to be pushed around the convention hall in a wheelchair. Bear in mind those dreadful injuries that she had had in her jump, and her debilitated lungs from the TB and smoking. So her body was giving out on her. It was steamy and hot and horrible. The air conditioning was up really high and she got a chill from the cold. She was met at the airport, they got her off the plane, got her a wheelchair and wheeled her around the convention hall. She was really just so excited. I never did hear about it because I was supposed to pick her up the following Tuesday morning to take her up to Yale where she was going to see an eye specialist. She had that business, you know, with the dry eyes. Her tear ducts were clogged and she was going up to see what course of treatment she could have for that; she had seen a local GP in Eastern Connecticut where she lived. He gave her an antibiotic and told her to stay in bed, which she did. She sounded much better when I talked to her the next day and she said, "Well, I'll tell you all about New Orleans in the car when we drive up to New Haven." I said, "Oh good, I can't wait."

That night she made herself a little snack of sliced tomatoes and a cup of tea. Evidently, when she went to pour the hot water into the teacup, that's when she suffered the cerebral hemorrhage. She fell, and she was found the next morning by the housekeeper unconscious. She was rushed to the hospital. I got the call that Monday morning not to come, Marty was in the hospital, in critical condition. She died that evening. That was July 21 of 1980. So I never heard the details of the convention. I did hear, from people who were there, that it was stupendous; that she was stupendous, that she was radiant and looked better than she had looked in years. I was just dumbstruck because she was just so vital that even though she was older there was certainly nothing wrong with her mind, it was just that her body, which had taken such a battering, was gradually weakening. After a time I thought, you know, that was a terrific way to go. She probably never knew what hit her. She had come home filled with all the old fire and enthusiasm and excitement and had lived long enough to see her wildest dreams realized. The dream that she articulated back in the early forties out in Cleveland when she said, "Wouldn't it be something if someday there were rooms like this all over the country?" had come true.

October 1990

Where to Go for Help

Alcoholics Anonymous is listed in the phone book. A.A. exists in virtually every city in the world. When you call A.A., someone will take your name and, within minutes, a recovering alcoholic will call you back and talk to you.

For information about A.A. you can write to A.A. World Headquarters at:

Alcoholics Anonymous
Post Office Box 459
Grand Central Station, New York, NY 10163–1100
212–686–1100

Women for Sobriety is an alternative to A.A., although some women use both programs—or, as Jean Kirkpatrick said, "Now women have three choices. They can use A.A., A.A. *and* W.F.S., or just W.F.S., whereas before they only had one choice: A.A." When you call W.F.S., Jean or someone else from W.F.S. will talk to you, send you information, and help you find a group that meets in your area. For more information about Women for Sobriety call:

215–536–8026

or write:

Women for Sobriety
P.O. Box 618
Quakertown, PA 18951

If you are concerned about a family member you can find Al-Anon in the phone book, or write:

Al-Anon Family Group Headquarters
P.O. Box 862
Midtown Station
New York, NY 10018–0862
212–302–7240

If you are interested in attending an Adult Children of Alcoholics meeting, call Alcoholics Anonymous or write:

National Association for Children of Alcoholics
31582 Coast Highway, Suite B
So. Laguna, CA 92677–3044

Another source of information on alcoholism:

National Council on Alcoholism and Drug Dependence
12 W. 21st Street, 7th Floor
New York, NY 10010
212–206–6770

If you are a heavy drinker but are unsure about whether or not you are an alcoholic, you might want to take the test Marty Mann developed. You must not stop drinking altogether; any alcoholic can do that. When you drink, have at least one drink and no more than three. If you drink every day then try the above every day. If you do not drink every day, perform the test on the days you do drink. Try this for at least six months. If you never exceed three drinks, chances are you are not an alcoholic. If you exceed the three drinks, even once, you have flunked the test. Alcoholics who try this test find that they are miserable with just three drinks. Stopping altogether is almost painless compared with taking one to three drinks a day. "Heavy drinkers" easily pass the test.

Or you may wish to take the following test, developed by the National Council on Alcoholism and Drug Dependence. Put a "yes" or a "no" next to each question:

1. Do you occasionally drink heavily after an appointment, a quarrel, or when the boss gives you a hard time?
2. When you have trouble or feel under pressure, do you always drink more heavily than usual?
3. Have you noticed that you are able to handle more liquor than you did when you were first drinking?
4. Did you ever wake up on the morning after and discover that you could not remember part of the evening before, even though your friends tell you that you did not pass out?

5. When drinking with other people, do you try to have a few extra drinks when others will not know it?

6. Are there certain occasions when you feel uncomfortable if alcohol is not available?

7. Have you recently noticed that when you begin drinking you are in more of a hurry to get the first drink than you used to be?

8. Do you sometimes feel a little guilty about your drinking?

9. Are you secretly irritated when your family or friends discuss your drinking?

10. Have you recently noticed an increase in the frequency of your memory "blackouts"?

11. Do you often find that you wish to continue drinking after your friends say they have had enough?

12. Do you usually have a reason for the occasions when you drink heavily?

13. When you are sober, do you often regret things you have done or said while drinking?

14. Have you tried switching brands or following different plans for controlling your drinking?

15. Have you often failed to keep promises you have made to yourself about controlling or cutting down on your drinking?

16. Have you ever tried to control your drinking by making a change in jobs or moving to a new location?

17. Do you try to avoid family or close friends while you are drinking?

18. Are you having an increasing number of financial and work problems?

19. Do more people seem to be treating you unfairly without good reason?

20. Do you eat very little or irregularly when you are drinking?

21. Do you sometimes have the shakes in the morning and find that it helps to have a few drinks?

22. Have you recently noticed that you cannot drink as much as you once did?

23. Do you sometimes stay drunk for several days at a time?

24. Do you sometimes feel very depressed and feel life is not worth living?

25. Sometimes after periods of drinking, do you see or hear things that are not there?

26. Do you get terribly frightened after you have been drinking heavily?

"Yes" answers to questions 1–8 indicate the early stages of alcoholism;

"yes" answers to 9–21 indicate the middle stages; "yes" answers to 22–26 indicate the final stages of alcoholism.

FURTHER READING

Nonfiction

I have found the following books invaluable:

Hobe, Phyllis. *Lovebound: Recovering from an Alcoholic Family*. New York: Penguin, 1990.
Kirkpatrick, Jean. *Goodbye Hangovers, Hello Life: Self-Help for Women*. New York: Ballantine, 1987.
Kirkpatrick, Jean. *Turnabout: Help for a New Life*. Quakertown, PA: Women for Sobriety, 1978.
Mann, Marty. *Marty Mann Answers Your Questions About Drinking and Alcoholism*. New York: Holt, Rinehart and Winston, 1970.
Mann, Marty. *Marty Mann's New Primer on Alcoholism*. New York: Holt, Rinehart and Winston, 1981.
Peele, Stanton. *The Diseasing of America: Addiction Treatment Out of Control*. Boston: Lexington Books, 1989.
Robertson, Nan. *Getting Better: Inside Alcoholics Anonymous*. New York: Fawcett, 1989.
Vaillant, George E. *The Natural History of Alcoholism*. Cambridge, MA: Harvard University Press, 1983.
Wholey, Dennis. *The Courage to Change*. New York: Warner Books, 1984.

Fiction and Autobiographies

Benedict, Elizabeth. *The Beginner's Book of Dreams*. New York: Knopf, 1988.
Duras, Marguerite. *The Lover*. Translated from the French by Barbara Bray. New York: Random House, 1985.
Fitzgerald, F. Scott. *Tender Is the Night*. New York: Macmillan, 1985.
Kirkland, Gelsey. *Dancing On My Grave*. New York: Jove Publications, 1987.
Lamott, Anne. *Rosie*. Berkeley, CA: North Point Press, 1983.
London, Jack. *John Barleycorn, Or Alcoholic Memoirs*. New York: Penguin, 1990.
McFarland, Dennis. *The Music Room*. New York: Avon, 1991.
McMillan, Terry. *Disappearing Acts*. New York: Penguin, 1989.

Roth, Philip. *The Facts: A Novelist's Autobiography*. New York: Penguin, 1989.

Sexton, Linda Gray. *Rituals*. New York: Doubleday, 1982.

Smith, Betty. *A Tree Grows in Brooklyn*. New York: Harper and Row, 1968.

Styron, William. *Set This House on Fire*. New York: Random House, 1960.

The Twelve Steps of Alcoholics Anonymous

1. We admitted that we were powerless over alcohol—that our lives had become unmanageable.
2. Came to believe that a power greater than ourselves could restore us to sanity.
3. Made a decision to turn our will and our lives over to the care of God *as we understood Him.*
4. Made a searching and fearless moral inventory of ourselves.
5. Admitted to God, to ourselves, and to another human being the exact nature of our wrongs.
6. Were entirely ready to have God remove all these defects of character.
7. Humbly asked Him to remove our shortcomings.
8. Made a list of all persons we had harmed, and became willing to make amends to them all.
9. Made direct amends to such people wherever possible, except when to do so would injure them or others.
10. Continued to take personal inventory and when we were wrong promptly admitted it.
11. Sought through power and meditation to improve our conscious contact with God *as we understood him,* praying only for knowledge of His will for us and the power to carry that out.
12. As a result of these steps, we tried to carry this message to alcoholics, and to practice these principles in all our affairs.

These are the original steps, as they were written by Bill Wilson.

The Thirteen Affirmations of Women for Sobriety

1. I have a life-threatening problem that once had me.
2. Negative emotions destroy only myself.
3. Happiness is a habit I will develop.
4. Problems bother me only to the degree I permit them to.
5. I am what I think.
6. Life can be ordinary or it can be great.
7. Love can change the course of my world.
8. The fundamental object of life is emotional and spiritual growth.
9. The past is gone forever.
10. All love given returns.
11. Enthusiasm is my daily exercise.
12. I am a competent woman and have much to give life.
13. I am responsible for myself and for my actions.

Glossary

Active. Still drinking.

Adult Children of Alcoholics (ACOA). Adults who were raised by an alcoholic parent(s).

Al-Anon. The program for friends and relatives of alcoholics, it was founded by Lois Wilson. Al-Anon helps family members cope with the stress of living with an alcoholic. It addresses the "disease" known as codependency. Many alcoholics join Al-Anon because they find themselves in relationships with other alcoholics.

Antabuse (disulfiram). A small white pill, this medication is used to ensure a person won't be tempted to drink. A few of the side effects of alcohol taken concurrently with Antabuse are vomiting, flushing of the skin, and in some instances death. Many people feel that by taking Antabuse they only have to make one decision, *not to drink*, rather than a hundred decisions, *"Should I drink?"*

Back out, or Go back out. Using drugs or alcohol again; it can also mean leaving the A.A. program to "go back out" and drink.

Big Book. The nickname for *Alcoholics Anonymous*.

Blacking out. Not to be confused with passing out; blacking out is "not remembering" what happened when one was under the influence, but still awake and functioning. It is a form of amnesia.

Bottom. High bottom, low bottom. These terms define how far down a person goes before recovery. "I hit bottom when . . . "

Codependency. The "disease" relatives and friends develop from living with an alcoholic. Al-Anon addresses the problems of codependency.

Coin. A coin the size of a half-dollar, it is given to A.A. members upon anniversaries, thirty, sixty, and ninety days of sobriety, and in treatment centers after successful completion.

Copping. "Getting" drugs.

Denial. The inability to accept that you are an alcoholic. Alcoholism is sometimes referred to as "a disease of denial."

Dry. Someone who has stopped drinking, but still feels miserable.

EAP. Employee Assistance Program. Designed to help employees with chemical dependencies.

Eightball. An eighth of an ounce of cocaine.

Enabling. Anything that helps the alcoholic to continue drinking, such as calling an employer to explain the alcoholic is "sick," or bailing the alcoholic out of jail.

Fox, Dr. Ruth. A psychiatrist who successfully treated many alcoholics. She introduced Antabuse (disulfiram) to this country. She was not an alcoholic.

Freebasing. Cooking and smoking cocaine.

N.A. Narcotics Anonymous.

Out there. Drinking or drugging.

Picking up. Using drugs.

Program. A.A., N.A., W.F.S.

Smith, Dr. Bob. A co-founder of Alcoholics Anonymous.

Speedballing. A mixture of cocaine and heroin.

Steps. The twelve steps of Alcoholics Anonymous.

White chip. A plastic disc the size of a half-dollar given to newcomers and people who have relapsed or slipped and come back into Alcoholics Anonymous.

White-knuckling. Using willpower to stop drinking.

Wilson, Bill. One of the co-founders of Alcoholics Anonymous.

Yets. A term used in Alcoholics Anonymous similar to "I told you so." When people say, "I never lost a job," a typical response would be, "not yet."

ABOUT THE AUTHOR

SARAH HAFNER is a writer and artist. She is also a recovering alcoholic. She lives in Northampton, Massachusetts, where she is currently at work on her second book.